Clinical Cases in Dermatology

Series Editor
Robert A. Norman, Tampa, USA

This series of concise practical guides is designed to facilitate the clinical decision-making process by reviewing a number of cases and defining the various diagnostic and management decisions open to clinicians.

Each title is illustrated and diverse in scope, enabling the reader to obtain relevant clinical information regarding both standard and unusual cases in a rapid, easy to digest format. Each focuses on one disease or patient group, and includes common cases to allow readers to know they are doing things right if they follow the case guidelines.

Antonella Tosti • Brian W Morrison
Torello Lotti
Editors

Clinical Cases in Nail Disorders

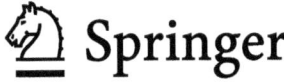 Springer

Editors
Antonella Tosti
Dr. Phillip Frost Department of
Dermatology and Cutaneous Surgery
University of Miami Miller School of
Medicine
Miami, FL, USA

Brian W Morrison
Dr. Phillip Frost Department of
Dermatology and Cutaneous Surgery
University of Miami Miller School of
Medicine
Miami, FL, USA

Torello Lotti
Department of Dermatology
University of Rome "G.Marconi"
Rome, Italy

ISSN 2730-6178   ISSN 2730-6186 (electronic)
Clinical Cases in Dermatology
ISBN 978-3-031-88641-6   ISBN 978-3-031-88642-3   (eBook)
https://doi.org/10.1007/978-3-031-88642-3

This Springer imprint is published by the registered company Springer Nature Switzerland AG
The registered company address is: Gewerbestrasse 11, 6330 Cham, Switzerland

If disposing of this product, please recycle the paper.

Contents

Chapter 1
Double Nail of the 5th Toe

Matilde Iorizzo ⓘ

Abstract Double nail of the 5th toe is a congenital anomaly where the nail plate splits into two parts, with the medial portion larger. Though not rare, it is underreported due to its often painless nature. Typically bilateral, it may involve toe rotation causing friction, thickening, and misdiagnosis as a callus. The condition is autosomal dominant, with no racial predisposition and a possible female predominance. Diagnosis is clinical, differentiating it from ectopic nails, fibrokeratoma, or traumatic deformities. Treatment is rarely needed but may involve surgical matricectomy or phenolization.

Keywords Nail dystrophy · Double nail · 5th toe abnormality · Matricectomy

Clinical Case Description

An otherwise healthy 10-year-old boy presented to the dermatologists with concerns regarding an unusual nail growth on his right and left 5th toe (Fig. 1.1). He reported discomfort but no pain. No significant medical history was reported, no history of trauma or injury to the affected toe.

The mother was particularly concerned about the presence of a wart, but this kind of infection has been promptly ruled out in both digits because upon dermoscopic examination there were no presence of typical mosaic pattern, colarette and dotted hemorrhages. The dermoscopic examination was able instead to reveal a nail plate splitted in two parts with the lateral part more dystrophic probably due to an extra rotation of the digit in a patient with splay feet (Fig. 1.2). There were no signs

M. Iorizzo (✉)
Private Dermatology Practice, Bellinzona/Lugano, Switzerland

© The Author(s), under exclusive license to Springer Nature
Switzerland AG 2025
A. Tosti et al. (eds.), *Clinical Cases in Nail Disorders*, Clinical Cases in
Dermatology, https://doi.org/10.1007/978-3-031-88642-3_1

1

Fig. 1.1 Clinical picture showing a dystrophic nail of the 5th toe

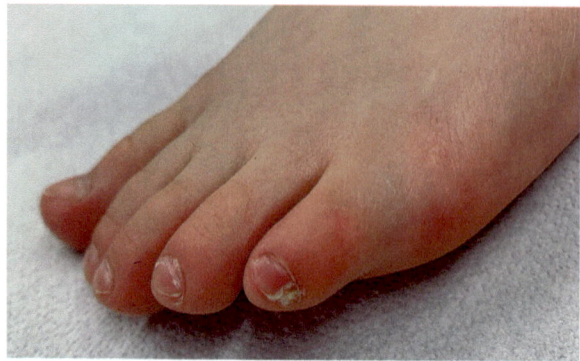

Fig. 1.2 Dermoscopy of the same nail presented in Fig. 1.1 showing a more detailed image of the condition: a double nail

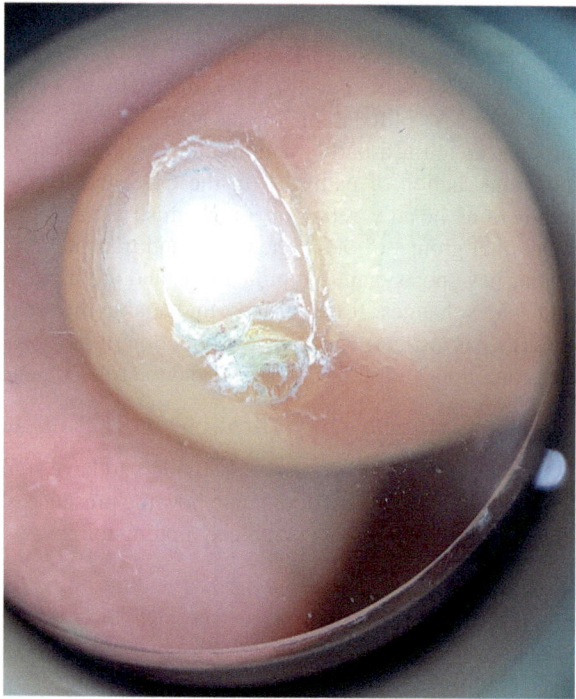

of inflammation, infection, or discharge surrounding the nail area. Given the non-inflammatory nature of the condition and absence of associated symptoms apart from occasional discomfort, conservative management options have been discussed with the patient and the mother that were additionally reassured regarding the benignity of the condition. Upon request the mother accepted to show her feet and a similar dystrophy has been detected in her 5th toenails also, gone unnoticed for many years.

What Is Your Diagnosis?

1. Double nail of the 5th toe
2. Ectopic nail
3. Nail spicule
4. FibrokeratomaThe correct diagnosis is double nail of the 5th toe.

Discussion

Based on the clinical presentation a diagnosis of the congenital anomaly known as double nail of the 5th toe was made. This condition is not rare, although rarely reported because often painless. Very often the problem is revealed during a foot examination done for other reasons because patients do not even realize they have nail dystrophy. The nail plate of the 5th toe, in affected patients, consists in two parts with the medial part bigger than the lateral one [1]. They are divided by a longitudinal depression or a real split [1]. The dystrophy is bilateral and in many cases the 5th digit is extra rotated with a subsequent friction on the lateral portion of the nail plate, the smaller one, which then becomes thicker, painful and can be misdiagnosed as a callus or a hard corn. This condition has been reported as autosomal dominant with multiple genes involved [2], females are mostly affected even if it is not clear if there is a gender prevalence. It is not a racial feature as it has been reported in many ethnicities.

The specific patient of the clinical case has not been investigated with an X ray because anything wouldn't have changed in terms of prognosis, but according to the literature a lazy Y at the tip of the distal phalanx or a Y-shaped tip as well as a thorn-like bony excrescence have been described [3]. There are however still many doubts on pathogenetic mechanisms – it is not clear yet, because never investigated, if this nail plate abnormality represents a very initial form of hexadactyly [3, 4]. To be noted the presence of a nail plate does not always require an underlying bone and vice versa. This condition should not be misdiagnosed as ectopic nail or fibrokeratoma [3, 4]. Ectopic nails are unusual in the feet and are not hereditary. However, they are detached nails and not the same splitted plate as in this case. They are also different from a histological point of view as ectopic nails presents a horizontal-vertical growth pattern and a distal or inverted orientation—the double nail of the 5th toe presents instead a horizontal-parallel growth pattern. A fibrokeratoma is a fibroepithelial lesion that forms in the periungual area or within or under the nail plate. It is a soft benign tumor easily distinguishable with a detailed clinical inspection. A traumatic double nail or a nail spicule from a wrong surgery can be ruled out taking the history of the patient. A callus or a wart can be easily ruled out with the aid of dermoscopy.

Most patients do not request treatment. However, for those who ask to remove the more dystrophic part of the plate, either phenolization of the accessory matrix or surgical matricectomy can be performed [3, 5]. In cases where histology has been performed, all components of the normal nail have been detected in the most pronounced cases and only an invagination of a thick hyperkeratotic epidermis with a broad stratum granulosum and a narrow cone of typical nail plate in the center in less pronounced cases with many intermediate instances [3].

Key Points

1. A rudimentary double nail of the 5th toe is not rare although rarely reported
2. This condition appears to be autosomal dominant with multiple genes involved
3. Treatment is not necessary and the decision is left to the patient

References

1. Hundeiker M. Hereditary dysplasia of the 5th toe. Hautarzt. 1969;20(6):281–2. German. PMID: 5355969
2. Srivastava P, Khunger N. A curious case of bilateral double fifth toenails: petaloid nails. Indian Dermatol Online J. 2023;14(4):556–7. https://doi.org/10.4103/idoj.idoj_444_22.
3. Haneke E. Double nail of the little toe. Skin Appendage Disord. 2016;1(4):163–7. https://doi.org/10.1159/000443378.
4. Ena P, Ena L, Ferrari M, Sotgiu MA, Mazzarello V. Double little toenails: report of 4 familial cases. JAAD Case Rep. 2020;6(4):365–8. https://doi.org/10.1016/j.jdcr.2020.02.008.
5. Chi CC, Wang SH. Inherited accessory nail of the fifth toe cured by surgical matricectomy. Dermatol Surg. 2004;30(8):1177–9. https://doi.org/10.1111/j.1524-4725.2004.30351.x.

Chapter 2
Drug-Induced Splinter Nail Haemorrhages in a Patient with Sézary Syndrome

Mirna Šitum, Nika Filipović Mioč, Mislav Mokos, and Vedrana Bulat

Abstract Splinter nail haemorrhages are thin, non-blanchable, longitudinal stripes beneath the nail plate that can appear red, brown, or black. Dermoscopic examination enhances visualization of these lines, which result from ruptured capillaries in the nail bed, with the blood integrating into the nail plate and moving distally as the nail grows. Common causes include trauma, skin and systemic diseases (e.g., psoriasis, connective tissue disorders), infections like endocarditis, and medication use.

This case report highlights a 72-year-old female with Sézary syndrome who developed drug-induced splinter nail haemorrhages following treatment with brentuximab vedotin. The patient initially presented with erythroderma, palmoplantar keratoderma, and lymphadenopathy, later progressing to stage IVB disease. Nail changes, manifesting as painful band-like longitudinal streaks on all nail plates, were observed after the 15th treatment cycle. These lesions, distinct from the broader nail changes typical of Sézary syndrome, correlated with the administration of brentuximab and advanced disease progression. The findings underscore the importance of monitoring nail lesions as potential markers of treatment efficacy and disease prognosis in Sézary syndrome.

Keywords Sézary syndrome · Splinter nail haemorrhages · Brentuximab vedotin · Drug-induced nail changes

M. Šitum · N. Filipović Mioč · M. Mokos (✉) · V. Bulat
Department of Dermatology and Venereology, Sestre milosrdnice University Hospital Center, Zagreb, Croatia
e-mail: mirna.situm@kbcsm.hr

A. Tosti et al. (eds.), *Clinical Cases in Nail Disorders*, Clinical Cases in Dermatology, https://doi.org/10.1007/978-3-031-88642-3_2

5

Clinical Case

A 72-year-old female presented to our department with erythroderma accompanied by intense pruritus, palmoplantar keratoderma and axillary lymphadenopathy. Her fingernails and toenails were affected by subungual hyperkeratosis and yellowish discolouration without subjective symptoms.

The patient had no history of previous dermatological diseases.

On admission, an elevated white blood count of 14,520/μL was noted (reference range 4,000–11,000/μL) with 55% lymphocytes. Flow cytometry revealed a high count of Sézary cells, measuring 4,700 cells/μL. Laboratory results included elevated lactate dehydrogenase (LDH) levels of 350 U/L (reference range, 135–214 U/L) and increased β2-microglobulin, recorded at 3.51 ng/L (reference range, ‹2.4 ng/L). The blood sample for HTLV-1 antibodies was negative.

Histopathologic findings of the affected skin revealed atypical lymphocytes within the epidermis, clustering to form Pautrier's microabscesses and dense, bandlike infiltrates within the dermis. Immunohistochemical staining showed CD4 and CD30 positivity (about 50%), with a noticeable absence of CD7+ (leu 9) cells. Histopathology of the enlarged axillary lymph node also showed dense accumulation of neoplastic T-cells, immunohistochemically positive for CD4 and CD30.

Peripheral flow cytometry indicated a dominant presence of CD4+ cells compared to CD8+ cells, with a ratio of 22:1. Clonal rearrangement of the T-cell receptor (TCR) β gene was observed in the skin, axillary lymph node, and blood. Positron emission tomography-computed tomography (PET-CT) scans of the chest, abdomen, and pelvis revealed multiple enlarged lymph nodes in both axillary and inguinal areas, with a maximum diameter of 2.4 cm and 1.7 cm, respectively. Mediastinal, abdominal, and pelvic lymph nodes were found to be within normal size limits (with diameters up to 0.8 cm).

As a result, the patient was diagnosed with stage IVA2 Sézary syndrome (T4N3M0B2). The patient underwent narrowband UV-B phototherapy in combination with topical steroids and Re-PUVA (a combination of a retinoid and 8 methoxypsoralen-UVA); however, these therapies did not produce a notable effect.

Therefore, brentuximab vedotin treatment was started at a dosage of 1.96 mg/kg in cycles spaced 30 days apart, without any other medication during this treatment. Brentuximab vedotin is a conjugate of an anti-CD30 antibody and monomethylauristatin E, which inhibits the polymerisation of microtubules. After completing 15 cycles, transverse linear brown bands accompanied with the nail plate depression appeared on the patient's fingernails and toenails. Within the bands, painful reddish-brown to black longitudinal streaks were noted (Fig. 2.1a). The tiny streaks and the disruption of the fine spiral arterioles within the nail bed were clearly visualised on dermoscopy.

Two weeks prior to the 15th treatment cycle, the patient's condition progressed to stage IVB (T4N3M1B2) Sézary syndrome, with substantial lymphocytosis and systemic involvement, including the spleen, liver, bone marrow, and nail matrices. The patient's white blood cell count, LDH, and β2-microglobulin levels were considerably raised, measuring 24,290/μL, 733 U/L, and 6.42 ng/L, respectively.

Following the 16th treatment cycle, the patient exhibited a second set of bandlike haemorrhages across all nail matrices (Fig. 2.1b), leading to the cessation of the therapy.

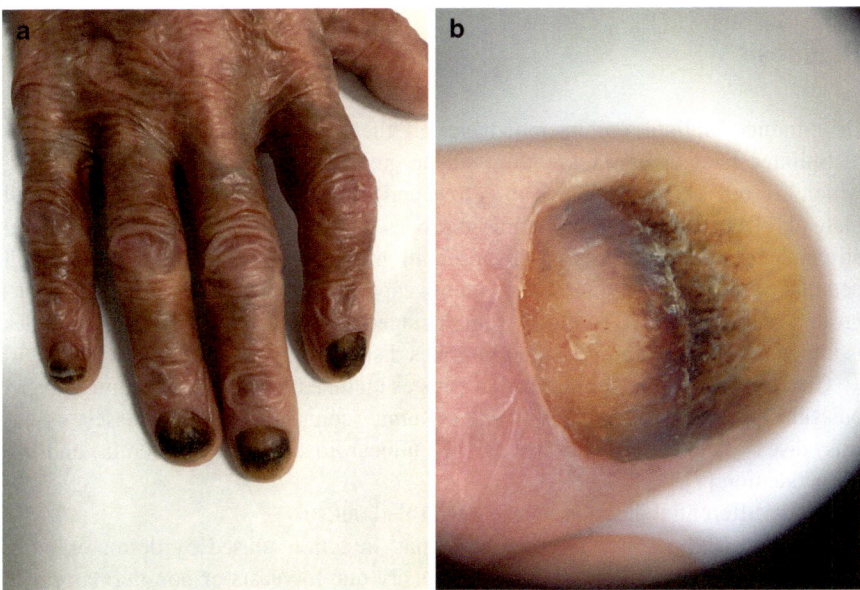

Fig. 2.1 Nail damage in a Sézary syndrome patient associated with brentuximab treatment. (**a**) Clinically, all nail plates on the hands and feet displayed a mixed pigmentation of yellow, red, and brown, accompanied by total disintegration of the distal half of the nail plate. (**b**) Sequential linear reddish-brown streaks observed on dermoscopy, accompanied by the nail plate depression: the lesions at the centre of the nail plate correspond to the 15th cycle, and those near the lunula are indicative of the 16th cycle of treatment

Based on the Case Description and the Photographs, What Is Your Diagnosis?

1. Onychomycosis
2. Trauma (subungual haemorrhage)
3. Drug-induced splinter nail haemorrhages
4. Connective tissue disease
5. Meningococcemia
6. Darier disease

Diagnosis

Drug-induced splinter nail haemorrhages are the correct diagnosis in this case.

Splinter haemorrhages are thin, linear, non-blanchable, longitudinal stripes, which are red, brown, or black in colour and usually located underneath the nail plate [1]. Dermoscopic examination improves the visualisation of the longitudinal alignment of red lines, enabling the observation of capillary dilations within the nail bed that occur before rupture. The ruptured capillaries of the dermis are in the background of this disease. The blood from damaged, longitudinally oriented capillaries is integrated into the nail plate and migrates distally along with nail growth.

Generally, causes of splinter haemorrhages include trauma (most common), various skin (psoriasis, lichen planus) and systemic (connective tissue diseases, vasculitis) diseases, infectious diseases (acute endocarditis, meningococcemia) and use of medication [1].

Other differential diagnoses have been ruled out.

Onychomycosis (*tinea unguium*) is a nail infection caused by dermatophytes. Less than 10% of cases of onychomycosis are due to yeasts or non-dermatophyte moulds [2]. The nails become discoloured (whitish to yellowish discoloration) and distorted (subungual hyperkeratosis). Several non-dermatophyte moulds, such as *Scopulariopsis brevicaulis* and *Scytalidium dimidiatum*, may cause brown and black discolouration of the nails. They initially invade the nail bed in the region of the hyponychium and eventually involve the entire nail bed and plate. Dermoscopy reveals an irregular brown or black band accompanied by thick subungual hyperkeratosis featuring yellow and brown scales. A novel dermoscopic pattern of subungual hyperkeratosis, referred to as a "ruin appearance," has recently been described, indicating the presence of fungal infection. Additionally, yellowish-white streaks within the matte black pigmentation can be found. The black pigmentation is wider at the distal edge than at the proximal edge, referred to as the "black reverse triangle". The distribution of lesions in onychomycosis is usually limited to one or several digits, as opposed to this case, where all of the nail plates were involved. Potassium hydroxide examination and cultivation in Sabouraud dextrose agar help to differentiate onychomycosis from other conditions [1].

Trauma is a very common cause of subungual nail haemorrhage (blood leaks from arterioles between the nail matrix and nail plate). Subungual nail haemorrhage mostly affects a single nail of the dominant hand in an otherwise healthy individual, while all nails were involved in our patient. Subungual haemorrhage may be painless, tender, or painful, as opposed to this case, where splinter nail haemorrhages were extremely painful. Subungual haemorrhage is usually well-demarcated and may appear homogeneous or with variable colours (reddish, purple, brown, black) due to the duration and stage of haematoma *reabsorption*. The discolouration resolves slowly over months and migrates distally with nail growth. A clear proximal margin in the nail plate (the starting point of nail formation) appears within a few weeks due to normal nail growth after the injury. In the case of temporary uncertainty in disease diagnosis, the nail should be monitored using dermoscopy. The prominent purplish globular structures (also known as dots) adjacent to the lesion with peripheral fading can be observed on dermoscopy [1].

Connective tissue diseases (CTD) can affect nails in many ways but most commonly affect the proximal nail fold capillaries. Alterations in capillary morphology within the proximal nail fold are predominantly linked to systemic lupus erythematosus (SLE), systemic sclerosis (SSc), and dermatomyositis (DM) but may also occur in mixed connective tissue disease (MCTD) and Sjögren's syndrome. Two distinct patterns of capillary telangiectasias in this region, observable through dermoscopy, indicate specific CTD. The first pattern, associated with SLE, is characterised by normal capillary density and irregular, meandering capillary loops. The second pattern, indicative of SSc or DM, is distinguished by reduced capillary density, dilated megacapillaries, neoangiogenic capillary loops, and extensive avascular areas. Microvascular lesions from different phases could be found in different nail fold areas in the same patient. Other nail lesions that can occur in CTD include subungual splinter haemorrhages, alterations in the thickness of the nail plates, and transverse curvatures in the fingernails. It has been shown that splinter haemorrhages occur more commonly in SLE, rheumatoid arthritis, SSc and DM than in healthy individuals [3]. Moreover, splinter haemorrhages in fingernails are associated with the activity of the disease in SLE, while transverse curvatures in fingernails indicate disease activity in SSc. Dermoscopy of the distal edge of the nail helps differentiate thickening of the nail due to nail plate thickening from thickening due to subungual hyperkeratosis. Furthermore, a red lunula (most commonly on fingernails) and transverse leukonychia (dermoscopically visible as white transverse bands within the nail plate) have been observed in patients with SLE. Additionally, in SSc, brittle nails are found as an indicator of increased nail plate fragility. In our patient, besides the absence of characteristic lesions on the proximal nail fold, which are expected in most patients with CTDs, the clinical picture of erythroderma cannot be associated with CTDs [1].

Meningococcaemia is etiologically linked to *Neisseria meningitidis*. The disease's heterogeneous acute clinical manifestations are attributable to its propensity for inducing diffuse endovascular damage. Pathophysiologically, meningococcaemia is characterised by widespread vascular injury, encompassing endothelial cell necrosis, intraluminal thrombosis, and perivascular haemorrhagic events. The initial clinical presentation of meningococcal disease may be nonspecific, characterised by a prodromal phase with symptoms such as cough, cephalalgia, and pharyngodynia. This prodrome may progress after a few days of upper respiratory tract symptoms, with an acute pyretic response often following a chilling sensation. Generalised asthenia, myalgia, cephalalgia, nausea, emesis, and arthralgia are typical initial symptoms. Meningococcemia may present initially with sparse, poorly defined cutaneous lesions, rapidly progressing to extensive petechial rash. In severe cases or fulminant meningococcaemia, patients may exhibit haemorrhagic skin eruptions, marked hypotension, myocardial depression, and swift augmentation of petechiae and purpuric lesions. Other dermatological symptoms, such as subungual splinter haemorrhages, have also been reported, especially in chronic meningococcaemia. The confirmatory diagnosis of meningococcal infection necessitates the isolation and culture of the causative organism, *Neisseria meningitidis*, from blood, cerebrospinal fluid, synovial fluid, or occasionally cutaneous lesions. Since our patient had neither the clinical signs nor laboratory results that could indicate meningococcaemia, this diagnosis has been ruled out [1, 2].

Darier's disease (follicular dyskeratosis) is inherited in an autosomal dominant pattern, and its leading cause lies in the mutation of the ATP2A2 gene, which encodes for the enzyme SarcoEndoplasmic Reticulum Calcium-ATPase (SERCA2) that is required to transport calcium within the keratinocytes. Patients usually present with numerous pruritic keratotic papules on the skin of seborrheic and intertriginous areas. Firmly adhering grey to brown-yellow hyperkeratosis can be found adjacent to the papules. The papules can form larger plaques, which may be covered with greasy crusts. Most patients with Darier disease will have multiple, alternating longitudinal broad red and white streaks within the nail plate of several or all fingernails. These nail lesions might mimic nail haemorrhages, but the detection of a V-shaped indentation of the distal nail margin is very suggestive of Darier disease. Onychoscopy is in accordance with the clinical presentation: splinter haemorrhages are commonly associated with digital ravines on the nail plate; additionally, alternating red and white streaks are better visualised and may be linked to the thinning of the nail plate. Nail lesions do not improve with oral retinoid therapy. A subungual benign tumour (onychopapilloma) might present as a single red longitudinal band (longitudinal erythronychia) and this sign is not sufficient to diagnose Darier disease. Darier disease is diagnosed by its clinical features and family history. Diagnosis may require a skin biopsy. Histopathological analysis reveals acanthosis, parakeratosis, dyskeratotic, eosinophilic cells in the spinous layer (corps ronds), and parakeratotic and dyskeratotic cells in both the granular and the corneal layer (grains) [2].

Based on the patient's medical history, clinical picture, and dermoscopy, the diagnosis of drug-induced splinter nail haemorrhages was made.

Of note, drug-induced splinter nail haemorrhages might be associated with decreased efficacy of the drug in patients with advanced Sézary syndrome, and these patients should therefore be subjected to regular oncologic follow-ups.

Discussion

Sézary syndrome is a type of cutaneous T-cell lymphoma (CTCL) that occurs due to the malignant growth of central memory T-cells. It is marked by erythroderma, generalised lymphadenopathy, and the presence of circulating neoplastic T cells with abnormally convoluted, cerebriform nuclei known as Sézary cells. The diagnostic criteria for Sézary syndrome include identifying an increased population of CD4+ T-cells leading to a CD4+ to CD8+ ratio greater than 10 and/or abnormal expression of pan-T-cell antigens, along with a minimum count of 1,000 Sézary cells/μL [4]. Ideally, the same T-cell clone should be detected in the peripheral blood, skin, and lymph nodes. Clinically, this syndrome manifests with intense itching and thickened, reddish skin, particularly on the face (*facies leonina*), with severe scaling, ectropion, hair loss, palmoplantar keratoderma, and onychodystrophy. The nail changes can include a variety of nonspecific features, such as subungual hyperkeratosis, yellowish discolouration of the nails, onycholysis, horizontal indentations on the nails (Beau's lines), paronychia, leukonychia, onychomadesis, and twenty-nail dystrophy [5].

Our patient met all the above-mentioned diagnostic criteria for Sézary syndrome. Upon admission, her nail lesions were nonspecific and consisted of painless subungual hyperkeratosis and yellowish discoloration of the nails without any evidence of bleeding. However, following the treatment with brentuximab, new lesions appeared on all fingernails and toenails in the form of painful band-like splinter haemorrhages.

Brentuximab vedotin consists of a chimeric IgG1 antibody targeting CD30, linked covalently to monomethyl auristatin E. This compound attaches to tubulin, inhibiting its polymerisation and consequently disrupting the microtubule network [6].

Brentuximab has been employed for treating Sézary syndrome in our patient because of its ability to specifically target malignant CD30+ T-cells, which were predominantly present in our patient's peripheral blood, lymph nodes, and skin [6].

During the initial two months of treatment, the patient experienced a swift improvement in her skin condition, and her blood parameters returned to normal. However, two weeks prior to the 15th treatment cycle, the disease advanced to stage IVB (T4N3M1B2). This progression was characterised by substantial lymphocytosis and widespread involvement of the spleen and liver, as well as infiltration into the bone marrow.

Following 15 cycles of treatment, the patient developed painful bandlike splinter haemorrhages on all fingernails and toenails, along with damage to the delicate spiral arteries within the nail bed. The emergence of nail lesions coincided with a marked increase in the number of Sézary cells in the peripheral blood, the bone marrow, and nail matrices.

Following the 16th round of treatment, the patient exhibited a second set of bandlike haemorrhages across all nail matrices. The prescribed information notes that brentuximab has a half-life of 4–6 days in humans, which might account for the absence of nail lesions in the intervals between consecutive brentuximab treatments [7]. The longitudinal growth of the nails offers a precise understanding of the impact of brentuximab on the malignant CD30+ T lymphocytes, as illustrated in Fig. 2.1.

So far, several cases of drug-induced splinter nail haemorrhage have been described in the literature, most associated with multi-kinase inhibitors like sunitinib and sorafenib. These agents, known for their antiangiogenic properties, disrupt the reparative processes of capillaries within the nail bed following trauma. Notably, such haemorrhages are observed in approximately 60–70% of patients undergoing treatment with kinase inhibitors, serving as a clinical indicator of the drugs' antiangiogenic activity.

Furthermore, various other pharmacological agents have been implicated in the aetiology of splinter nail haemorrhages. These include nitrofurantoin, ganciclovir, tetracycline hydrochloride, and terbinafine [8]. Moreover, the emergence of targeted antineoplastic therapies, such as cabozantinib and those inhibiting vascular endothelial growth factor receptor (VEGFR), has been associated with the induction of splinter subungual haemorrhages. The onset of splinter haemorrhages is often temporally correlated with initiating treatment involving VEGFR inhibitors. These haemorrhages typically manifest during the initial weeks of therapy and are noted to resolve spontaneously. The natural progression of the nail growth leads to the gradual outward movement of these haemorrhages, effectively diminishing their visibility over time. It is considered that inhibition of VEGFR plays a significant role in restricting the physiological repair mechanisms of nail bed capillaries [1]. In the exceedingly uncommon instances where Sézary syndrome is accompanied by nail haemorrhages, these typically affect the whole nail plate. This contrasts with our patient, whose lesions exhibited a distinct sequential pattern. This pattern can be linked to the monthly administration of brentuximab and its direct cytotoxic impact on the CD30+ T lymphocytes in the nail matrix [9].

It is important to note that splinter nail haemorrhages in our patient, besides being associated with brentuximab therapy, may also be linked to the progression of the underlying disease, as documented two weeks before the onset of these nail lesions. Therefore, these nail changes have been considered a significant adverse event and an indicator of an unfavourable prognosis. This state is in line with the opinion of Bishop et al., who suggest that nail alterations might serve as valuable indicators in evaluating the efficacy of systemic treatments [10]. However, to ascertain the prognostic value of nail haemorrhages induced by brentuximab in patients with advanced stages of Sézary syndrome, more comprehensive studies and further research are needed [10].

We anticipate that our findings will prompt medical professionals to give greater consideration to nail lesions in patients with Sézary syndrome, as these could offer crucial information for future studies of the condition.

Key Points

1. This case study highlights splinter nail haemorrhages as an adverse event linked to brentuximab.
2. Nail haemorrhages caused by brentuximab display clinical differences from typical nail lesions seen in Sézary syndrome, which generally affect the entire nail plate. In contrast, the lesions in this instance exhibit a distinct pattern correlating with the monthly administration of brentuximab.
3. Nail haemorrhages induced by brentuximab could be indicative of reduced effectiveness of the drug in patients suffering from advanced stages of Sézary syndrome.

References

1. Baran R. Advances in nail disease and management. Springer; 2021. https://doi.org/10.1007/978-3-030-59997-3.
2. Plewig G, French L, Ruzicka T, Kaufmann R, Hertl M. Braun-Falco's dermatology. 4th ed. Berlin/Heidelberg: Springer; 2022. https://doi.org/10.1007/978-3-662-63709-8.
3. Tunc SE, Ertam I, Pirildar T, Turk T, Ozturk M, Doganavsargil E. Nail changes in connective tissue diseases: do nail changes provide clues for the diagnosis? J Eur Acad Dermatol Venereol. 2007;21(4):497–503. https://doi.org/10.1111/j.1468-3083.2006.02012.x.
4. Kamijo H, Miyagaki T. Mycosis Fungoides and Sézary syndrome: updates and review of current therapy. Curr Treat Options Oncol. 2021;22(2):10. https://doi.org/10.1007/s11864-020-00809-w.
5. Park K, Reed J, Talpur R, et al. Nail irregularities associated with Sézary syndrome. Cutis. 2019;103(4):E11–6.
6. Mehra T, Ikenberg K, Moos RM, et al. Brentuximab as a treatment for CD30+ mycosis fungoides and Sézary syndrome. JAMA Dermatol. 2015;151(1):73–7. https://doi.org/10.1001/jamadermatol.2014.1629.
7. Bradley AM, Devine M, DeRemer D. Brentuximab vedotin: an anti-CD30 antibody-drug conjugate. Am J Health Syst Pharm. 2013;70(7):589–97. https://doi.org/10.2146/ajhp110608.
8. Haber R, Khoury R, Kechichian E, Tomb R. Splinter hemorrhages of the nails: a systematic review of clinical features and associated conditions. Int J Dermatol. 2016;55(12):1304–10. https://doi.org/10.1111/ijd.13347.
9. Damasco FM, Geskin LJ, Akilov OE. Nail changes in Sézary syndrome: a single-center study and review of the literature. J Cutan Med Surg. 2019;23(4):380–7. https://doi.org/10.1177/1203475419839937.
10. Bishop BE, Wulkan A, Kerdel F, et al. Nail alterations in cutaneous T-cell lymphoma: a case series and review of nail manifestations. Skin Appendage Disord. 2015;1(2):82–6. https://doi.org/10.1159/000433474.

Chapter 3
Nail Changes Associated with Chronic Graft-Versus-Host Disease

Eun Jae Kim ⓘ **and Jennifer Huang** ⓘ

Abstract Nail dystrophy is an underrecognized manifestation of lung involvement in chronic graft-versus-host disease (cGVHD) in children. We present a case of a 17-year-old male with a history of allogeneic bone marrow transplant who developed nail dystrophy 17 months post-transplant in the context of lung cGVHD. Clinical findings included polydactylous longitudinal erythronychia, onychorrhexis, and distal nail splitting. Management of cGVHD-associated nail dystrophy is primarily symptom-driven. This case highlights the importance of routine nail examinations in patients with cGVHD.

Keywords Graft-versus-host disease · Bone marrow transplant · Onychorrhexis · Erythronychia · Prognosis

Case Summary

A 17-year-old male with a history of refractory mixed phenotype acute leukemia underwent treatment with allogeneic bone marrow transplant. Seven months after his bone marrow transplant, he developed severe multi-organ graft-versus-host disease (GVHD) involving the gastrointestinal tract, liver, eyes, oral mucosa, and skin. Initial skin involvement included a pruritic, macular rash involving the arms, chest,

E. J. Kim
Harvard Medical School, Boston, MA, USA
e-mail: eunjaekim@hms.harvard.edu

J. Huang (✉)
Harvard Medical School, Boston, MA, USA

Boston Children's Hospital, Boston, MA, USA
e-mail: Jennifer.huang@childrens.harvard.edu

© The Author(s), under exclusive license to Springer Nature
Switzerland AG 2025
A. Tosti et al. (eds.), *Clinical Cases in Nail Disorders*, Clinical Cases in
Dermatology, https://doi.org/10.1007/978-3-031-88642-3_3

15

back and dorsal feet. No sclerotic or lichenoid features were noted. All clinical symptoms of GVHD, including that of the skin, initially improved with his first course of oral steroids, ruxolitinib, and vedolizumab. However, with the tapering of his oral steroids, he developed transaminitis and mild color and textural changes of the skin that were concerning for liver and cutaneous chronic GVHD (cGVHD). Mildly decreased forced expiratory volume (FEV1) was also noted on pulmonary function test (PFT) at 15 months post-transplant. Given no clear pattern of restrictive or obstructive lung disease, the change was attributed to deconditioning, and the oncology care team decided to monitor with serial PFTs. Both liver and cutaneous cGVHD improved with another course of oral steroids, and the patient was continued on long-term immunosuppressive treatment with ruxolitinib and interleukin-2 injections.

The patient presented to dermatology at 17 months post-transplant for follow up of his cutaneous cGVHD. At this visit, patient reported no recent skin flares or concerns. A complete cutaneous examination revealed multiple bands of longitudinal red streaks and ridging involving multiple fingernails (Fig. 3.1). Distal splitting was also noted on the right thumb nail plate (Fig. 3.2). The patient reported no pain or discomfort associated with the nail changes, and he was unsure of their chronicity. There were no signs of cutaneous cGVHD aside from residual hyperpigmented macules of the face, trunk, and arms. Nail matrix biopsy was deferred at this visit, and no treatments were prescribed for his nail dystrophy given their asymptomatic nature.

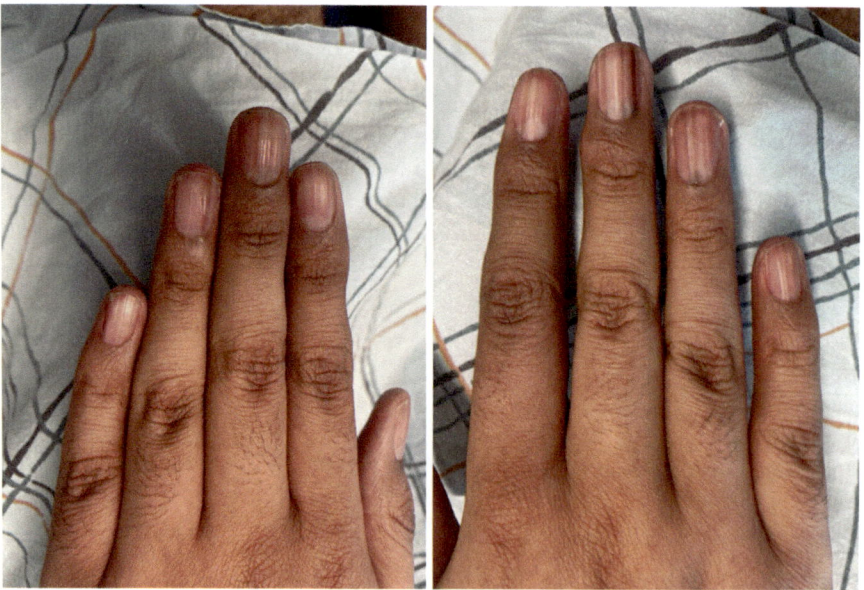

Fig. 3.1 Longitudinal erythronychia and onychorrhexis involving multiple digits of the hands

Fig. 3.2 Distal nail splitting of the right thumb

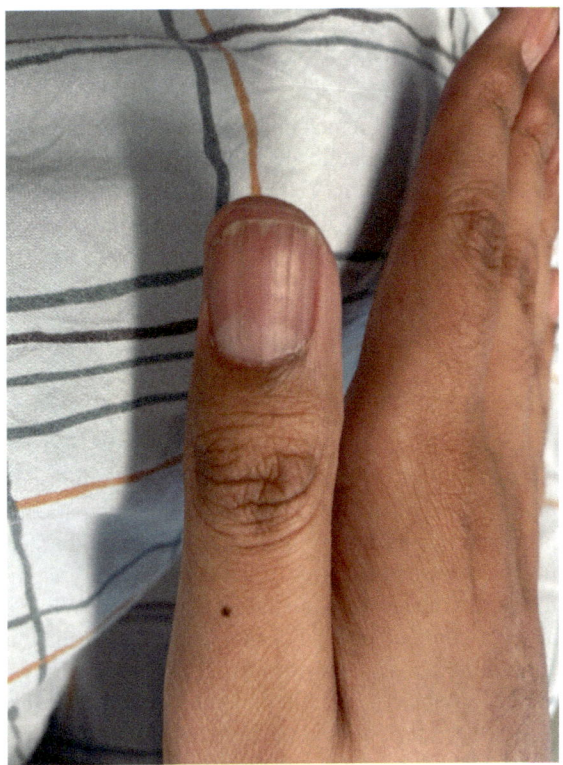

Two months later, patient underwent his next routine PFT, which revealed a significantly decreased FEV1 of 58%. A few weeks later, patient presented to the emergency room with chest pain and dyspnea. Chest CT revealed air trapping with bronchiectasis, and lung biopsy revealed patchy alveolar damage and absent bronchioles suggestive of pulmonary cGVHD. His clinical symptoms improved with a course of oral steroids, montelukast, azithromycin, inhale fluticasone. His PFTs remained consistent with a nonreversible obstructive pattern.

The patient was seen 4 years later with an new history of an asymptomatic red and brown rash involving his face and trunk. On physical exam, he had multiple violaceous plaques involving the face, chest, abdomen, and back. Exam of the plaques under dermoscopy revealed white reticulated lines consistent with Wickham's striae. Nail exam appeared stable from prior, with longitudinal red streaks, ridging, and distal nail splitting involving multiple digits of the hand. Patient was diagnosed with lichenoid cutaneous cGVHD and treated with topical tacrolimus 0.1% ointment and triamcinolone 0.1% ointment.

Diagnosis

Differential for the etiology of the patient's polydactylous longitudinal erythronychia (red streaks) included cGVHD, lichen planus, other multifocal inflammatory
diseases, and idiopathic [1, 2]. Onychorrhexis (ridging) is associated with systemic
conditions such as cGVHD, systemic amyloidosis, rheumatoid arthritis, and nutritional deficiency [3]. Based on patient's medical history and lack of other skin or
systemic findings, his nail dystrophy was determined to be a harbinger of
lung cGVHD.

Discussion

Chronic graft-versus-host disease is a common complication of allogeneic bone
marrow transplant that significantly impacts patient morbidity and mortality [4]. It
is caused by an immune reaction between donor stem cells and host tissues. Organ
involvement and severity of cGVHD can vary significantly between patients, and
the skin is the most frequently affected organ. While cutaneous cGVHD is tradition-
ally classified as either lichenoid or sclerodermatous, skin involvement can range
from mild xerosis to erythroderma [5]. Adnexal involvement is also common, with
nail dystrophy observed in up to half of patients with cutaneous cGVHD [6].

Our patient presented with onychorrhexis, erythronychia and distal nail splitting,
all of which are known nail changes associated with cGVHD [5–7]. Onychorrhexis
refers to longitudinal ridging on the superficial layer of the nail. It is the most common nail change seen in patients with cutaneous cGVHD [6, 7]. Longitudinal erythronychia refers to linear red band(s) on the nail plate originating from the proximal
nail fold. Distal nail splitting often occurs concurrently with erythronychia due to
thinning of the nail bed. Other nail changes that may occur in setting of cGVHD
include periungual telangiectasia, pterygium, onycholysis, periungual erythema,
and textural changes of the nail [6, 7].

Pathogenesis of the various nail manifestations in patients with cGVHD is poorly
understood. Lichenoid infiltration of nail matrix may be responsible for some
cGVHD-associated nail dystrophy; nail changes seen with cGVHD closely resemble lichen planus-associated nail dystrophy and often occur in the context of lichenoid cutaneous cGVHD [1, 8, 9]. In one reported case of an adult transplant patient
with nail thickening, fragility, onycholysis, longitudinal striations, and pterygium,
nail biopsy revealed a lichenoid pattern [8]. However, some patients with nail dystrophy have sclerodermatous rather than lichenoid form of cGVHD, suggesting that
nail dystrophy could be caused by multiple pathways [6, 7]. Our patient initially
presented with nail dystrophy without other signs of active cutaneous cGVHD but
developed lichenoid cutaneous cGVHD several years later.

Nail exams are crucial to perform in all patients with cGVHD because nail dystrophy may portend severe cGVHD. In one cohort study of children with cGVHD,

nail dystrophy was associated with steroid-resistant cGVHD, sclerotic cGVHD, and lung cGVHD [7]. In our patient, nail dystrophy preceded his diagnosis of lung cGVHD. Given that his PFT had been declining prior to the development of his nail dystrophy, our patient likely had progressive pulmonary cGVHD that remained undiagnosed and untreated until the patient became symptomatic. Pulmonary function should be closely monitored in patients with nail dystrophy for timely work up of lung cGVHD.

Management of cGVHD-associated nail dystrophy is primarily symptom-driven. Oral supplementation with vitamins, in particular biotin (vitamin B7), can improve nail fragility [10]. Commercially available nail strengtheners or nail moisturizers can also be recommended. The underlying cGVHD should be appropriately treated in patients with evidence of active cGVHD.

Key Points

- Nail manifestations of chronic graft-versus-host disease (cGVHD) include onychorrhexis, erythronychia, distal splitting, periungual telangiectasia, pterygium, onycholysis, periungual erythema, and textural changes.
- Conducting nail exams for all patients with cGVHD is essential as nail dystrophy may portend severe cGVHD, including steroid resistant disease, sclerotic skin involvement, and/or lung cGVHD.

References

1. Cohen PR. Longitudinal erythronychia: individual or multiple linear red bands of the nail plate: a review of clinical features and associated conditions. Am J Clin Dermatol. 2011;12(4):217–31. https://doi.org/10.2165/11586910-000000000-00000.
2. Jellinek NJ. Longitudinal erythronychia: suggestions for evaluation and management. J Am Acad Dermatol. 2011;64(1):167.e1–167.e11. https://doi.org/10.1016/j.jaad.2009.10.047.
3. Singal A, Arora R. Nail as a window of systemic diseases. Indian Dermatol Online J. 2015;6(2):67–74. https://doi.org/10.4103/2229-5178.153002.
4. Zecca M, Prete A, Rondelli R, et al. Chronic graft-versus-host disease in children: incidence, risk factors, and impact on outcome. Blood. 2002;100(4):1192–200. https://doi.org/10.1182/blood-2001-11-0059.
5. Hymes SR, Turner ML, Champlin RE, Couriel DR. Cutaneous manifestations of chronic graft-versus-host disease. Biol Blood Marrow Transplant. 2006;12(11):1101–13. https://doi.org/10.1016/j.bbmt.2006.08.043.
6. Sanli H, Arat M, Oskay T, Gürman G. Evaluation of nail involvement in patients with chronic cutaneous graft versus host disease: a single-center study from Turkey. Int J Dermatol. 2004;43(3):176–80. https://doi.org/10.1111/j.1365-4632.2004.01629.x.
7. Huang JT, Duncan CN, Boyer D, Khosravi H, Lehmann LE, Saavedra A. Nail dystrophy, edema, and eosinophilia: harbingers of severe chronic GVHD of the skin in children. Bone Marrow Transplant. 2014;49(12):1521–7. https://doi.org/10.1038/bmt.2014.194.

8. Palencia SI, Rodríguez-Peralto JL, Castaño E, Vanaclocha F, Iglesias L. Lichenoid nail changes as sole external manifestation of graft vs. host disease. Int J Dermatol. 2002;41(1):44–5. https://doi.org/10.1046/j.0011-9059.2001.01399.x.

9. Liddle BJ, Cowan MA. Lichen planus-like eruption and nail changes in a patient with graft-versus-host disease. Br J Dermatol. 1990;122(6):841–3. https://doi.org/10.1111/j.1365-2133.1990.tb06280.x.

10. Chessa MA, Iorizzo M, Richert B, et al. Pathogenesis, clinical signs and treatment recommendations in brittle nails: a review. Dermatol Ther. 2020;10(1):15–27. https://doi.org/10.1007/s13555-019-00338-x.

Chapter 4
Secondary Raynaud's Phenomenon with Gangrene in the Setting of Systemic Sclerosis

Heather Gochnauer, Priscilla Romano, Elizabeth Rainone, Ruth Ann Vleugels, and Diana Reusch

Abstract Systemic sclerosis associated with secondary Raynaud's phenomenon and digital ulceration can be treated with botulinum toxin injections.

Keywords Systemic sclerosis · Raynaud's phenomenon · Digital ulceration · Gangrene · Botulinum toxin

Clinical Case

An eleven-year-old girl presented with a seven-year history of pain in her fingers, worsened by cold exposure. Physical exam (Fig. 4.1) was notable for distal finger skin tightness and slight tapering. Fingertips had a violaceous hue. There was hyperkeratosis at the hyponychium of all ten fingernails, consistent with pterygium inversum unguis. The right fourth finger and left fourth finger had superficial, dry

Co-first authors: Drs. Heather Gochnauer and Priscilla Romano.

H. Gochnauer · P. Romano
Division of Pediatric and Adolescent Dermatology, Rady Children's Hospital San Diego, San Diego, California, USA
Department of Dermatology, University of Massachusetts Chan Medical School, Worcester, MA, USA
e-mail: Hgochnauer@health.ucsd.edu; Priscilla.romano@umassmemorial.org

E. Rainone · R. A. Vleugels
Department of Dermatology, Brigham and Women's Hospital, Harvard Medical School, Boston, MA, USA
e-mail: erainone@bwh.harvard.edu; rvleugels@bwh.harvard.edu

D. Reusch (✉)
Department of Dermatology and Pediatrics, University of Massachusetts Chan Medical School, Worcester, MA, USA
e-mail: Diana.reusch@umassmemorial.org

© The Author(s), under exclusive license to Springer Nature Switzerland AG 2025
A. Tosti et al. (eds.), *Clinical Cases in Nail Disorders*, Clinical Cases in Dermatology, https://doi.org/10.1007/978-3-031-88642-3_4

Fig. 4.1 Palmar hands showing distal skin tightness, violaceous hue of fingertips, and finger tapering. Hyperkeratosis at the hyponychium of the nails consistent with pterygium inversum unguis. Right fourth finger and left fourth finger superficial, dry erosions. Right second distal fingertip gangrenous change. Left third distal fingerpad pitting. Left fourth and fifth fingers with absent lunulae and slightly increased curvature (Left third fingernail with nail polish proximally)

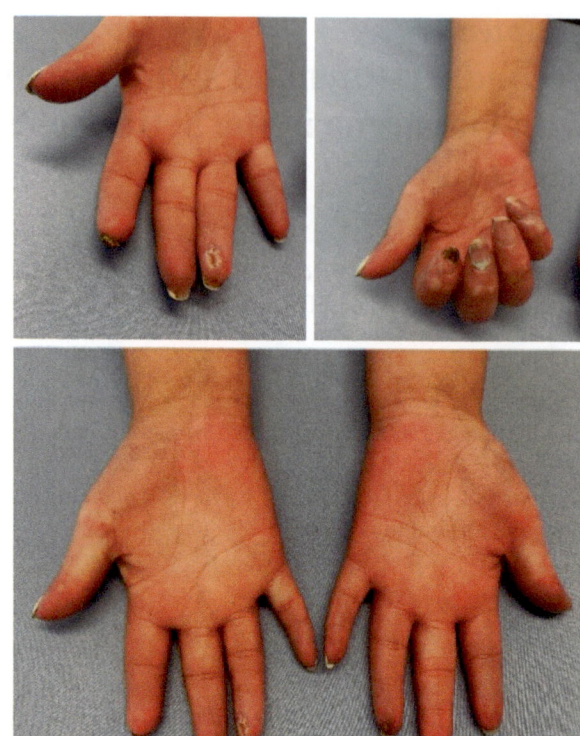

erosions and the right second distal fingertip had gangrenous change. Laboratory work-up revealed positive ANA at 1:1280 (speckled pattern) and SCL-70 IgG elevated to 252. Antibodies to RNP, histone, CCP, Ro, La, centromere, RF, and dsDNA were all negative. ESR was within normal limits. CT chest showed mild interstitial lung disease. Nuclear medicine esophageal and esophageal nanometer were normal, though the patient experienced symptoms of gastroesophageal reflux disease. Echocardiogram was normal.

Pain persisted despite behavioral modifications to keep her core and extremities warm. Trialed and failed medications included amlodipine, aspirin, hydroxychloroquine, fluoxetine, mycophenolate mofetil, nifedipine, pentoxifylline, prednisone, sildenafil, and tocilizumab. Given persistence of her symptoms despite numerous therapies, botulinum toxin injections to the neurovascular bundle of each finger were initiated, with symptom improvement and healing of her right second finger gangrenous ulcer.

Based on the Case Description and the Photographs, What Is Your Diagnosis?

- Systemic lupus erythematosus
- Dermatomyositis
- Juvenile idiopathic arthritis
- Systemic sclerosis
- Infection

Diagnosis

Systemic sclerosis.

Discussion

Systemic sclerosis (SSc, scleroderma) is a rheumatologic condition driven by underlying immune system activation, fibrosis, and vasculopathic changes affecting multiple organ systems.

Almost all patients with SSc (>96%) experience a secondary Raynaud's phenomenon (RP), which can predate other disease symptoms by years [1]. RP is a symmetric, vasospastic disorder that classically results in triphasic color change of the fingers and toes, is associated with uncomfortable sensory symptoms, and occurs in the absence of arterial occlusion [2]. RP begins as a reversible vasospasm due to functional changes in the digital arteries of the hands and feet. However, over time, many patients with SSc develop progressive structural changes in the small blood vessels that permanently impair flow [2]. 30–70% of SSc patients develop digital ulcerations (DU) [1], and those affected by DU are at risk of gangrene [3].

Nail changes are common in patients with systemic sclerosis, with 80.6% of patients affected in a prospective cohort of 129 French patients [4]. In this cohort, the presence of nail changes was significantly associated with digital ulceration, and there were specific nail abnormalities associated with digital ulcers. These included: thickened nails, scleronychia, brachyonychia, parrot beaking, hyponychium hyperkeratosis, pterygium unguis, splinter hemorrhages, and cuticular changes. Vasculopathy is presumed to be responsible for both digital ulcerations and as well as these nail changes in patients with SSc.

Other risk factors for digital ulceration in patients with SSc are early onset of RP, diffuse and early disease, anti-Scl70 antibodies present, and male sex (though SSc is overall more common in women) [5].

Treatment for SSc is typically determined by organ involvement and symptomatology. Methotrexate, mycophenolate mofetil, or azathioprine may be used to treat skin thickening [6]. Treatment options for RP include environmental interventions, such as keeping extremities and core warm with extra layers of clothing and avoiding smoking. PDE5 inhibitors (e.g., sildenafil, tadalafil) and calcium channel blockers (e.g., amlodipine, nifedipine) are first-line oral therapies. When these traditional treatment options fail, botulinum toxin A (BTX-A) is an effective treatment option [7–9]. BTX-A, a selective acetylcholine release inhibitor, is thought to improve digital blood flow and inhibit vasoconstriction via vascular smooth muscle paralysis and blocking of noradrenaline release [8]. Adjunctive treatment options include but are not limited to topical nitrate, angiotensin receptor blockers, or selective serotonin reuptake inhibitors. For digital ulcerations that do not respond to oral therapy or injected BTX-A, intravenous prostacyclin can be an effective rescue therapy [10].

Key Points

- Patients with systemic sclerosis may be affected by severe Raynaud's phenomenon, digital ulcerations, and gangrenous fingertip lesions.
- Nails are frequently abnormal in patients with SSc and the following changes are associated with digital ulceration: thickened nails, scleronychia, brachyonychia, parrot beaking, hyponychium hyperkeratosis, pterygium unguis, splinter hemorrhages, and cuticular changes.
- Botulinum toxin A injection is a well-tolerated, emerging therapy for severe, refractory Raynaud's phenomenon.

References

1. Meier FMP, Frommer KW, Dinser R, et al. Update on the profile of the EUSTAR cohort: an analysis of the EULAR scleroderma trials and research group database. Ann Rheum Dis. 2012;71:1355–60. https://doi.org/10.1136/annrheumdis-2011-200742.
2. Pauling JD, Hughes M, Pope JE. Raynaud's phenomenon—an updated on diagnosis, classification and management. Clin Rheumatol. 2019;38:3317–30. https://doi.org/10.1007/s10067-019-04745-5.
3. Mihai C, Distler O, Gheorghiu AM, et al. Incidence and risk factors for gangrene in patients with systemic sclerosis from the EUSTAR cohort. Rheumatology (Oxford). 2020;59(8):2016–23. https://doi.org/10.1093/rheumatology/kez558.
4. Marie I, Gremain V, Nassermadji K, et al. Nail involvement in systemic sclerosis. J Am Acad Dermatol. 2017;76(6):1115–23. https://doi.org/10.1016/j.jaad.2016.11.024.
5. Silva I, Almeida J, Vasconcelos C. A PRISMA-driven systematic review for predictive risk factors of digital ulcers in systemic sclerosis patients. Autoimmun Rev. 2015;14(2):140–52. https://doi.org/10.1016/j.autrev.2014.10.009. Epub 2014 Oct 14. PMID: 25449678
6. Kowal-Bielecka O, Fransen J, Avouac J, et al. Update of EULAR recommendations for the treatment of systemic sclerosis. Ann Rheum Dis. 2016;76(8):1327–39. https://doi.org/10.1136/annrheumdis-2016-209909.

7. Uppal L, Dhaliwal K, Butler PE. A prospective study of the use of botulinum toxin injections in the treatment of Raynaud's syndrome associated with scleroderma. J Hand Surg Eur. 2014;39(8):876–80. https://doi.org/10.1177/1753193413516242.
8. Barry KK, Reusch DB, Shahriari N, Lonowski S, Dedeoglu F, Vleugels RA. Botulinum toxin for refractory Raynaud's phenomenon: a "how to" guide for pediatric patients. Pediatr Dermatol. 2023;40(3):587–9. https://doi.org/10.1111/pde.15229.
9. Kassamali B, Desai S, Min M, et al. OnabotulinumtoxinA for systemic sclerosis-associated Raynaud's phenomenon: a multi-institutional study on accessibility and effectiveness. J Drugs Dermatol. 2021;20(11):1257–9. https://doi.org/10.36849/jdd.6135.
10. Sagonas I, Daoussis D. Treatment of digital ulcers in systemic sclerosis: recent developments and future perspectives. Clin Rheumatol. 2023;42(10):2589–99. https://doi.org/10.1007/s10067-023-06511-0.

Chapter 5
Onycholysis, Xantonychia and Melanonychia Due to *Nakaseomyces glabrata* (*Candida glabrata*)

Roberto Arenas (ID) and Eder R. Juárez-Durán (ID)

Abstract We report a male with diabetes mellitus and nail affection with onycholysis, chromonychia and paronychia. Dermoscopy showed lateral onycholysis with xantonychia and melanonychia. In mycological study *Nakaseomyces glabrata* was identified (formlery *Candida glabrata*). Onycholysis is common in woman and related with a broad spectrum of causes such as psoriasis or drugs. When associated with discoloration suggest the presence of *Candida* or *Trichosporon*. Xantonychia and melanonychia, can be observed in other nail diseases, but, when onycholysis is present, *Candida* is usually involved. Paronychia usually requires a mild-potency topical steroid in management.

Keywords *Candida glabrata* · Chromonychia · Melanonichia · Paronychia · Xantonychia

Clinical Case

We report a 66-year-old male school teacher, from Mexico City, with Type II diabetes mellitus in control with metformin.

He presented a nail disease affecting the right thumbnail with one-month history of lateral onycholysis with chromonychia and paronychia (Fig. 5.1). Dermoscopic test (medicam 800HD®—FotoFinder, Bad Birnbach) showed lateral onycholysis with xantonychia and melanonychia (Fig. 5.2).

R. Arenas (✉) · E. R. Juárez-Durán
"Dr. Manuel Gea González" General Hospital, México City, Mexico

© The Author(s), under exclusive license to Springer Nature Switzerland AG 2025
A. Tosti et al. (eds.), *Clinical Cases in Nail Disorders*, Clinical Cases in Dermatology, https://doi.org/10.1007/978-3-031-88642-3_5

Fig. 5.1 Close-up of a
thumb with a thickened,
discolored nail, possibly
indicating a fungal
infection

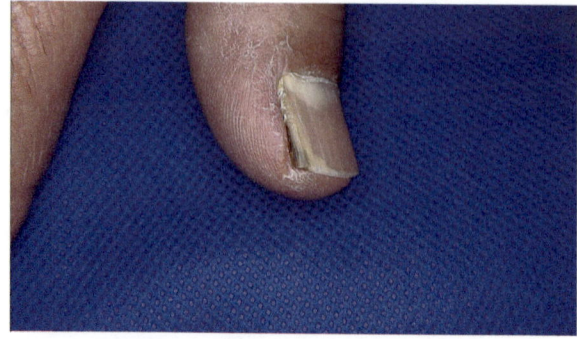

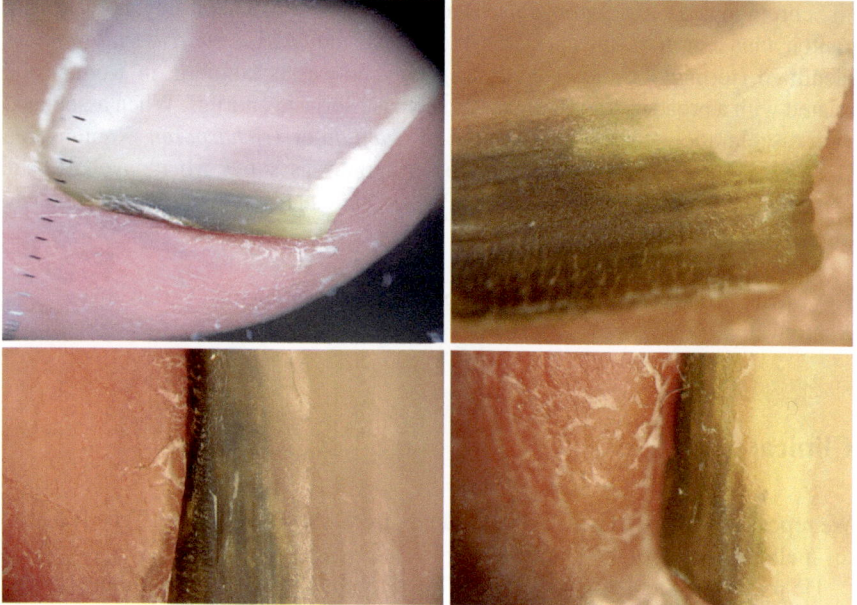

Fig. 5.2 Image of a fingernail with a green-brownish discoloration. Dermoscopy of the side of the
nail, highlighting the green-brownish streaks and texture of the surrounding skin

Differential Diagnosis

- Traumatic onycholisis
- Xantonychia and melanonychia
- Fungal onycholisis
- Onycholisis related to psoriasis

Laboratory Tests

Mycological study with KOH (chlorazol-Black®—Delasco, Council Bluffs) showed blastospores. *Candida* sp. was isolated in Sabouraud (BD, La pont de Clax) dextrose agar and the specie was identified with CHROMagar Candida® (BD, La pont de Clax): *Nakaseomyces glabrata* (formlery *Candida glabrata*).

Diagnosis

Onycholysis, xantonychia and melanonychia due to *Nakaseomyces glabrata* (C. *glabrata*).

Discussion

Onycholysis is a common condition in nail diseases observed in woman occurring mainly in fingernails. It consists in the distal separation of the plate from the nail bed, due to disruption of the so called onychocorneal band [1, 2]. Commonly related with a broad spectrum of causes such as psoriasis or drugs, also can be occupational and secondary to trauma, manicuring or self-induced. *Candida* sp. usually colonizes this onycholytic space (between the plate and the nail bed), more frequently by *C. albicans* and *C. parapsilosis,* sometimes this yeast has been recovered from the vaginal and gastrointestinal tract [3].

We are presenting an elderly male patient with diabetes as the only underlying condition and due to limited affection of the nail, onycholysis and discoloration, this can suggest the presence of *Candida* or *Trichosporon* infection. Fungal chromonychia is an infection due to dermatophytes, Non-dermatophyte molds or *Candida*, and when onycholysis is present, it becomes a predisposing factor for a yeast infection, especially *Candida* sp. [4]

Nail pigmentation or melanonychia can be due to melanocyte activation or melanocyte hyperplasia. It is more frequent in pigmented skin in Asian or African-Americans. Xantonychia or yellow discoloration could be a normal finding in elderly or secondary to jaundice, carotenes, tetracyclines, antimalarials, gold and other dermatological conditions including onychomycosis and psoriasis.

This case presents xantonychia and melanonychia, that can be observed in other dermatological-related nail diseases or even exogenous pigment, but when onycholysis is also present, *Candida* is usually involved [5, 6].

The goal of management in this case is to minimize trauma to the affected nail and, avoid water or irritant substances and aggressive self-cleaning of the nail bed; it is also recommended to wear cotton gloves under rubber gloves during manual work [7]. Additionally, remove the onycholytic nail every 2 weeks until the nail plate grows back normally; carefully clean and dry the nailbed before applying a topical antiseptic (2–4% thymol in chloroform or topical tretinoin 0.025% gel once a day) [8].

In nail fold inflammation or paronychia it usually requires a mild-potency topical steroid (methylprednisolone aceponate 0.1%), or tacrolimus 0.1% twice a day and in severe cases systemic steroids (methylprednisone 20 mg/ kg/d) or intralesional triamcinolone acetonide 2.5 mg/ml can be used [7].

Key Points

1. Onycholisis can be related to psoriasis, drugs or fungal infection (*Candida* sp), it can be also occupational and secondary to trauma
2. Melanonychia can be due to melanocyte activation or melanocyte hyperplasia and related to several conditions including fungal infections
3. When suspecting a fungal infection, mycological test is mandatory

References

1. Daniel CR 3rd. Onycholysis: an overview. Semin Dermatol. 1991;10(1):34–40.
2. Daniel CR 3rd, Iorizzo M, Piraccini BM, Tosti A. Simple onycholysis. Cutis. 2011;87(5):226–8.
3. Zaias N, Escovar SX, Zaiac MN. Finger and toenail onycholysis. J Eur Acad Dermatol Venereol. 2015;29(5):848–53. https://doi.org/10.1111/jdv.12862. Epub 2014 Dec 16
4. Ortega-Springall MF, Arroyo-Escalante S, Arenas R. Onycholysis and Chromonychia: a case caused by *Trichosporon inkin*. Skin Appendage Disord. 2016;1(3):144–6. https://doi.org/10.1159/000441065. Epub 2015 Nov 24
5. Hyeon Bae S, Young Lee M, Lee JB. Distinct patterns and aetiology of chromonychia. Acta Derm Venereol. 2018;98(1):108–13. https://doi.org/10.2340/00015555-2798.
6. Mendiratta V, Jain Indian A. Nail dyschromias. J Dermatol Venereol Leprol. 2011;77(6):652–8. https://doi.org/10.4103/0378-6323.86473.
7. Iorizzo M. Tips to treat the 5 most common nail disorders: brittle nails, onycholysis, paronychia, psoriasis, onychomycosis. Dermatol Clin. 2015;33(2):175–83. https://doi.org/10.1016/j.det.2014.12.001.
8. Dias PCR, Miola AC, Miot HA. Successful management of chronic refractory onycholysis by partial nail avulsion followed by topical tretinoin. An Bras Dermatol. 2019;94(1):118–9.

Chapter 6
Onychomycosis in a Toddler Secondary to Thumb-Sucking

Eduardo Corona-Rodarte, Susana Landa-Horta, and Daniel Asz-Sigall

Abstract Onychomycosis in toddlers is an exceptionally rare condition, made even more unique by its association with behavioral habits like thumb-sucking. We present the case of a one-year-old male with persistent yellowish discoloration, onychodystrophy, and paronychia of both thumbnails. Dermoscopic findings, alongside culture results confirming *Candida albicans*, guided a successful treatment strategy using oral nystatin. This case underscores the critical role of behavioral factors in pediatric nail pathology and highlights the importance of integrating clinical, dermoscopic, and microbiological evidence for accurate diagnosis. This report elucidates an underrecognized pediatric presentation, contributing to a more comprehensive understanding of fungal nail infections and their management in early childhood.

Keywords Onychomycosis · Toddler · Thumb-sucking · *Candida albicans* · Pediatric nail infection

Clinical Case

A one-year-old male patient, previously healthy, presented to our dermatology clinic with a chief complaint of yellow discoloration of both thumbnails persisting for 4 months. The patient's parents reported that the discoloration began shortly after the onset of thumb-sucking behavior. Physical examination revealed yellowish discoloration, onychodystrophy, paronychia, and mild thickening of both thumbnails, with evidence of surrounding tenderness and erythema (Fig. 6.1). Dermoscopy revealed a ruin apperence and chromonychia with distal irregular termination (Fig. 6.2). The remaining nails appeared normal. Given these findings, a total dystrophic onychomycosis was suspected. A potassium hydroxide (KOH) preparation of nail clippings was performed, demonstrating fungal elements consistent with onychomycosis. The culture on Sabouraud's medium displayed smooth, white, and

E. Corona-Rodarte · S. Landa-Horta · D. Asz-Sigall (✉)
Trichology Unit, Hospital General "Dr. Manuel Gea González", Mexico City, Mexico

© The Author(s), under exclusive license to Springer Nature Switzerland AG 2025
A. Tosti et al. (eds.), *Clinical Cases in Nail Disorders*, Clinical Cases in Dermatology, https://doi.org/10.1007/978-3-031-88642-3_6

shiny colonies (Fig. 6.3). Additionally, the selective chromogenic medium revealed a green hue within 24 h, consistent with *Candida albicans*. Laboratory investigations ruled out underlying immunodeficiency or systemic illnesses predisposing to fungal infections. Oral nystatin was initiated, and the patient exhibited complete resolution over the subsequent months.

Relevant Figures

Fig. 6.1 Onychodystrophy, yellowish discoloration, paronychia, and mild thickening of both thumbnails

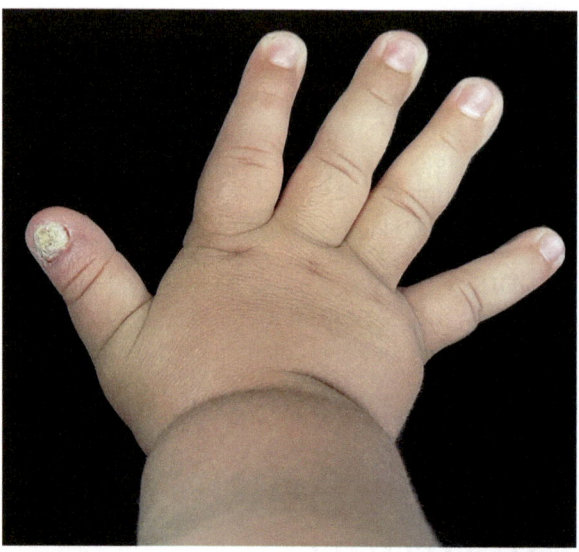

Fig. 6.2 Ventral indentations of the nail plate caused by dermal debris (ruin apperance), yellow discoloration (chromonychia), and distal pulverization of the nail plate (distal irregular termination)

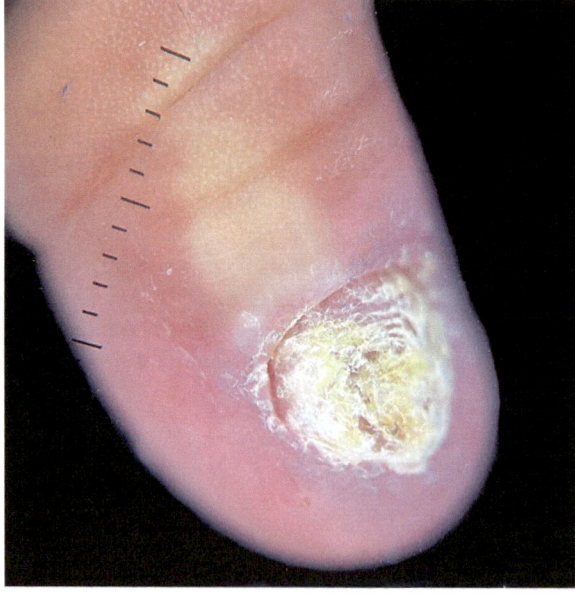

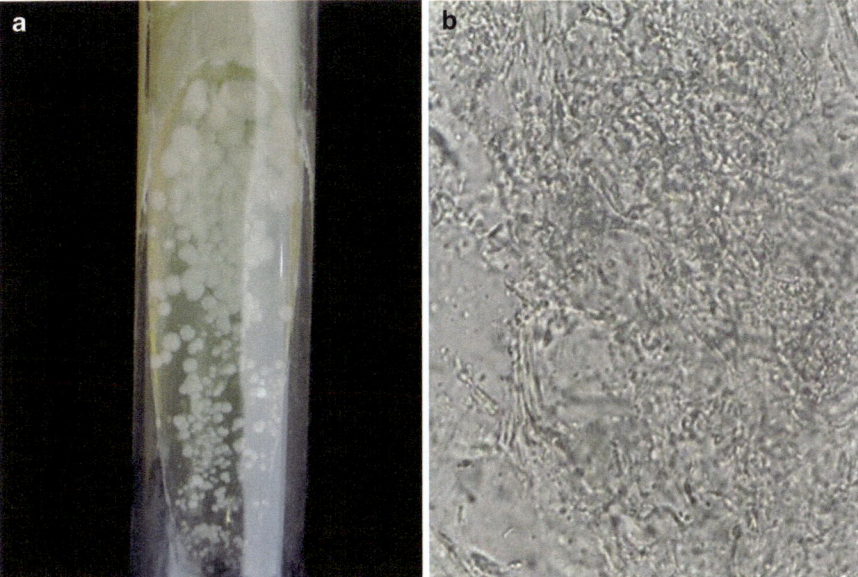

Fig. 6.3 Smooth, white, and shiny colonies on fungal culture (**a**). Microscopic visualization of fungal septae and hyphae on direct KOH testing (**b**)

Based on the Case Description and the Photographs, What Is Your Diagnosis?

- Onychomadesis
- Onychomycosis
- Nail psoriasis
- Nail trauma
- Lichen planus

Discussion

The presented case underscores the rarity of onychomycosis in toddlers, particularly in association with thumb-sucking behavior. Although fungal infections of the skin and nails are prevalent worldwide, their occurrence in pediatric populations, especially those under the age of two, remains uncommon. Our case highlights the significance of recognizing behavioral factors, such as thumb-sucking, in the etiology of nail infections in this age group.

The prevalence of onychomycosis in children is estimated to range from 0.2% to 2.6%, with variations observed across different geographical regions. While this prevalence is lower compared to adults, there is emerging evidence suggesting a rising incidence [1]. This increase may be attributed to factors such as the wide-spread use of occlusive footwear, participation in communal group activities, and evolving hygiene practices. Typically associated with advancing age, onychomycosis tends to manifest more frequently in older individuals. Several factors contribute to its relative rarity in children under the age of 16. These factors include differences in the structure of the nail plate, decreased susceptibility to trauma compared to adults, limited exposure to fungal pathogens in communal settings, and a lower incidence of concurrent tinea pedis infections [2].

Instances of onychomycosis in children under 2 years old are exceedingly rare, with documented risk factors including Down syndrome, immunosuppression, and perinatal hypoxia. Additionally, evidence suggests a genetic predisposition for Trichophyton rubrum (T. rubrum) infection in cases of distal subungual onychomycosis [3, 4]. Screening parents for superficial fungal infections is essential as they can potentially transmit the infection to their children.

Dermatophytes are often the primary isolated species in fungal nail infections, with T. rubrum being the most prevalent dermatophyte affecting both fingernails and toenails [5]. Onychomycosis tends to affect toenails more frequently than fingernails in children, especially in older age groups. In children under 6 years old, yeasts are commonly found in fingernail infections, possibly associated with behaviors such as finger sucking and a lower incidence of tinea pedis [6]. In cases of Candida spp. infections, onychodystrophy may be accompanied by perionyxis.

The most prevalent form of pediatric onychomycosis is distal and lateral subungual onychomycosis, characterized by yellow discoloration of the nail plate, subungual debris, onycholysis, and thickening of the distal and lateral nail plate areas [7]. These characteristic manifestations aid clinicians in promptly identifying and diagnosing the condition in pediatric patients. The list of potential differential diagnoses encompasses nail dystrophy resulting from various causes, including thumb malalignment, psoriasis, lichen planus, and alopecia areata.

Given the potential side effects associated with antifungal medications, it is essential to establish a definitive diagnosis before initiating treatment. Confirmation of the diagnosis requires the detection of fungi in a nail specimen through microscopic examination, culture, or other laboratory testing methods. Direct microscopic examination and fungal culture are considered the gold standard for diagnosing onychomycosis. A potassium hydroxide (KOH) preparation is often preferred due to its rapid availability of results, relatively low cost, and simplicity. However, it's crucial to note that the sensitivity of KOH preparation is lower compared to histopathologic examination with periodic acid-Schiff stain or polymerase chain reaction (PCR) [8].

Histopathologic examination of nail clippings with a PAS stain is a straightforward procedure known for its high sensitivity in identifying fungal elements. Fungal culture conducted on Sabouraud's medium enables both identification and speciation of fungal infection, with high specificity (ranging from 83% to 100%), albeit limited sensitivity [9]. Additionally, PCR, a molecular technique allowing for rapid and highly specific amplification of DNA fragments, has emerged as a sensitive diagnostic tool for onychomycosis. However, its use is constrained by limited availability, as PCR testing may not be widely accessible in all healthcare settings.

Pediatric onychomycosis treatment may not always require systemic therapy, as topical treatments often yield superior results. Topical antifungal agents such as ciclopirox, efinaconazole, and tavaborole have been shown to be safe and effective in children. Additionally, systemic antifungal agents like terbinafine, itraconazole, and fluconazole, administered per weight, have demonstrated safety in children and are utilized off-label for treating pediatric onychomycosis, exhibiting high efficacy [10]. In our patient's case, systemic therapy with nystatin was employed due to Candida colonization of the oral cavity.

In conclusion, while onychomycosis remains unrecognized in pediatric populations, clinicians should maintain a high index of suspicion, especially in the presence of predisposing factors such as thumb-sucking behavior. Early recognition and appropriate management are paramount in achieving successful outcomes and preventing potential complications in this vulnerable patient population.

Key Points

- Onychomycosis in children is potentially underreported, despite emerging evidence indicating an increasing incidence. Onychomycosis tends to manifest more frequently in older individuals, with a lower incidence in children under the age of 16.
- Dermatophytes, particularly *Trichophyton rubrum*, are commonly isolated in fungal nail infections, with yeasts more prevalent in younger children.
- Treatment approaches in pediatric onychomycosis may differ from adult cases, often involving topical antifungal agents as the first-line therapy and systemic agents administered off-label based on weight.

References

1. Solís-Arias MP, García-Romero MT. Onychomycosis in children. A review. Int J Dermatol. 2017;56(2):123–30. https://doi.org/10.1111/ijd.13392.
2. Bonifaz A, Saúl A, Mena C, et al. Dermatophyte onychomycosis in children under 2 years of age: experience of 16 cases. J Eur Acad Dermatol Venereol. 2007;21(1):115–7. https://doi.org/10.1111/j.1468-3083.2006.01802.x.
3. Zaias N, Tosti A, Rebell G, et al. Autosomal dominant pattern of distal subungual onychomycosis caused by Trichophyton rubrum. J Am Acad Dermatol. 1996;34(2 Pt 1):302–4. https://doi.org/10.1016/s0190-9622(96)80142-3.
4. García-Romero MT, Granados J, Vega-Memije ME, Arenas R. Analysis of genetic polymorphism of the HLA-B and HLA-DR loci in patients with dermatophytic onychomycosis and in their first-degree relatives. Actas Dermosifiliogr. 2012;103(1):59–62. https://doi.org/10.1016/j.adengl.2011.03.017.

5. Rodríguez-Pazos L, Pereiro-Ferreirós MM, Pereiro M Jr, Toribio J. Onychomycosis observed in children over a 20-year period. Mycoses. 2011;54(5):450–3. https://doi.org/10.1111/j.1439-0507.2010.01878.x.
6. Vestergaard-Jensen S, Mansouri A, Jensen LH, Jemec GBE, Saunte DML. Systematic review of the prevalence of onychomycosis in children. Pediatr Dermatol. 2022;39(6):855–65. https://doi.org/10.1111/pde.15100.
7. Song G, Zhang M, Liu W, Liang G. Children onychomycosis, a neglected dermatophytosis: a retrospective study of epidemiology and treatment. Mycoses. 2023;66(5):448–54. https://doi.org/10.1111/myc.13571.
8. Ameen M, Lear JT, Madan V, Mohd Mustapa MF, Richardson M. British Association of Dermatologists' guidelines for the management of onychomycosis 2014. Br J Dermatol. 2014;171(5):937–58. https://doi.org/10.1111/bjd.133584.
9. Lipner SR, Scher RK. Onychomycosis: clinical overview and diagnosis. J Am Acad Dermatol. 2019;80(4):835–51. https://doi.org/10.1016/j.jaad.2018.03.062.
10. Gupta AK, Venkataraman M, Shear NH, Piguet V. Onychomycosis in children – review on treatment and management strategies. J Dermatolog Treat. 2022;33(3):1213–24. https://doi.org/10.1080/09546634.2020.1810607.

Chapter 7
Frictional Subungual Hematoma of Both Big Toes

Patricia Chang (ID), **Gabriela Alarcon** (ID), **and Marisol Gramajo**

Abstract Subungual hematoma is the most common injury and cause of nail discoloration, which manifest itself as the accumulation of blood under the nail plate. It originates due to a strong blow or repetitive microtrauma to the distal phalanx, some of the frictional sbungual hematoma are due repetitive mirotrauma as the anatomy of the toes, use of shoes with narrow or steel toes, occupation, sports, recent use of oximeter. Any methods of blood detection can be used, such as urine strip test or fecal occult blood test.

Keywords Frictional subungual hematoma · Trauma · Nail discoloration · Urine test strip · Nail abnormalities · Nail disease · Pigmentation

Abbreviations

KOH   Potassium hydroxide

Clinical Case

A 77-year-old female patient was sent to our clinic for a second opinion due to the presence of a 3-year history of discoloration in the nails of both big toes of the feet, without associated symptoms. Patient reported that she has consulted multiple

P. Chang (✉)
Paseo Plaza Clinic Center, Guatemala City, Guatemala

G. Alarcon
Private Practice, Guatemala City, Guatemala

M. Gramajo
Hospital General de Enfermedades IGSS, Guatemala City, Guatemala

Fig. 7.1 Panoramic view
of both big toenails

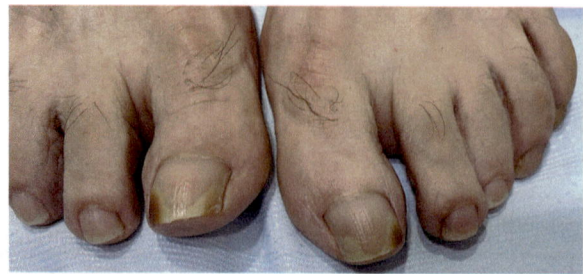

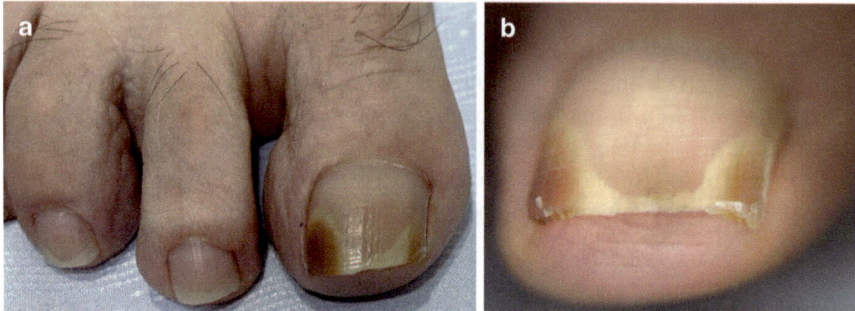

Fig. 7.2 (**a, b**) Onychoscopy showed nail discoloration and onycholysis in the right big toe

dermatologists due to the appearance of her nails, for which she had received multiple treatments with topical and systemic antifungals without obtaining any relief.

On physical examination, localized onychopathy was observed in the nails of both big toenails, consisting of onycholysis and reddish-brown discoloration (Fig. 7.1). On onychoscopy the reddish-brown coloration and onycholysis were accentuated (Figs. 7.2a, b and 7.3a, b), and on microscopy, a yellowish red coloration was observed in the nails (Fig. 7.4a, b).

Patient reported a medical history of Type 2 Diabetes Mellitus of 5 years duration, currently controlled with Metformin, 1000 milligrams orally once a day. He also reported a family history of a diabetic mother.

The diagnosis of Frictional subungual hematoma of both big toenails was done.

A urine strip test of sub-nail material, potassium hydroxide (KOH) test and culture for fungi and microscopy of the nails was indicated. The KOH and fungal culture were negative, serial sections of the nail under polarized light microscopy show hemorrhage on the inner surface of the nail, but the urine test strip showed the presence of blood in the subungual material (Fig. 7.5).

The patient was questioned again about a history of continuous blows or friction, and she recalled that her orthopedic surgeon instructed her to use shoe lifts, a time that coincides with the beginning of the alteration in nails color.

The patient was told to stop using the shoe lifts; unfortunately, we have not heard from her again.

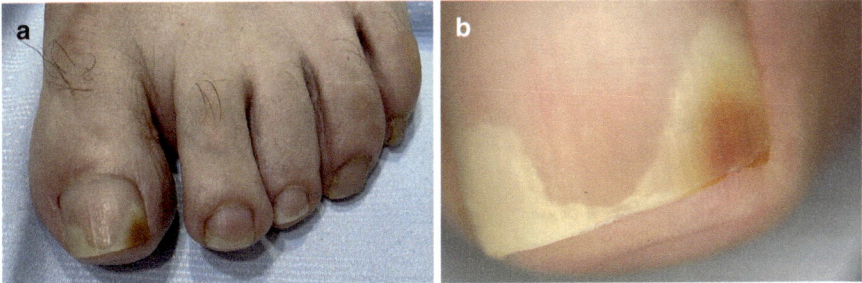

Fig. 7.3 (**a, b**) Onychoscopy showed nail discoloration and onycholysis in the left big toe

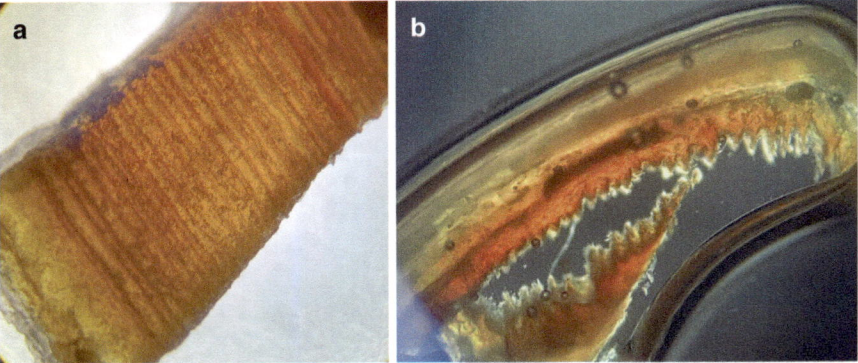

Fig. 7.4 (**a, b**) Serial sections of the nail under polarized light microscopy showed hemorrhage on the inner surface of the nail

Diagnosis and Relevant Differential Diagnosis Based on the Case Description and Photographs

Frictional Subungual Hematoma

Subungual hematoma is the most common injury and cause of nail discoloration, which manifest itself as the accumulation of blood under the nail plate. Depending on the evolution this can be acute and chronic; regarding location, they can affect hands and feet with predominancy in the first toes [1–4].

The most common subungual hematoma is the acute one, it originates due to a strong blow or repetitive microtrauma to the distal phalanx [4]. These injuries can be simple, when the nail and surrounding areas are preserved, and graves when there are important injuries such as fractures, avulsion due to crushing or loss of tissue. This type of hematoma generally manifest itself form small splinter hemorrhages to nail avulsion and is habitually accompanied by severe pain and swelling

Fig. 7.5 Urine test strip
showed the presence of
blood in the subungual
material

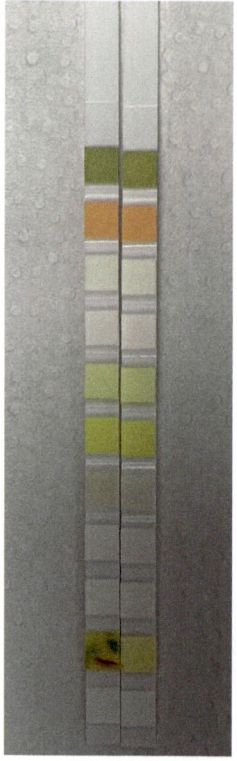

[3–5]. Treatment depends on the severity of the trauma, which is why different modalities have been proposed, such as simple observation, and the use of heated needles, nail avulsion, drills and lasers for trephining. These manifestations move distally according to the nail growth, so complete resolution is usually slow [1, 4, 5].

Frictional subungual hematoma also called chronic subungual hematoma, is caused by repetitive and continuous microtrauma to the nail. Its prevalence is grater in advanced ages and its most frequent location is the hallux; it can manifest bilaterally, symmetrically or unilaterally. This injury is common and usually goes unnoticed by patients since they normally do not present symptoms. In relation to its pathogenesis, it is important to take into account the anatomy of the toes, use of shoes with narrow or steel toes, occupation, sports, recent use of oximeter and concomitant diseases [2–6, 7]. On physical examination, it is usually observed as a brown-black dyschromia which can be partial, total or longitudinal, depending on the area of pressure exerted by the object in the nail [2–6, 8]. Onychoscopy shows the presence of a red-purple-brown pattern under the nail plate, homogeneous color and peripheral fading [2, 8, 9]. If there is doubt about the diagnosis, any methods of blood detection can be used, such as urine strip test or fecal occult blood test [4, 6, 7, 10].

Subungual Frictional Pseudohematoma

The subungual frictional pseudohematoma is a dyschromia caused by the accumulation of dirt propitiated by the lack of cleanliness of the nail. This entity can take on different colors and shapes such as linear, partial or total. It frequently occurs in older patients with difficulty in self-care of their nails. Furthermore, this entity is favored by concomitant diseases such as toe deformities and the use if inappropriate footwear. Diagnosis is based on physical examination and proper cleaning of the area [7]. Additionally, a test that rules out the presence of blood, can confirm the diagnosis [4, 6, 7, 10].

Frictional Melanonychia

The term melanonychia refers to the black, brown or gray pigmentation of the nail plate caused by the presence of melanin, due to the activation of melanocytes. This can vary in shape; however, it frequently appears as a longitudinal band that originates from the nail matrix to the distal edge, following the growth of the nail, the transverse and total forms are uncommon. Melanocytes in the nail matrix can be activated by inflammatory processes of the proximal nail fold, such as chronic exposure to friction, pressure and trauma. Frictional melanonychia most commonly affects the fifth and/or fourth toe, and it is not associated with abnormalities of the nail plate [8, 9]. The diagnosis can be made through onychoscopy which reveals a black-gray band with a brown background and fine parallel lines. Red spots or splinter hemorrhages may be present if there is damage to the capillaries [2, 8, 9].

Fungal Melanonychia

Fungal melanonychia is a very rare variant of onychomycosis, it is caused by direct melanin production by the fungi. *Trichophyton rubrum*, the most common pathogen, and *Scytalidium dimidiatum*, produce pigmented hyphae which can cause nail pigmentation. This pathology is common in older adults, appears primarily in the toe nails and usually affects a single nail unit. Onychoscopy reveals multicolored pigmentation, reverse triangular patterns, subungual hyperkeratosis, scales and yellowish-brown spots; in addition, no melanin inclusions are observed, which supports the non-melanocytic origin of the pigmentation [2, 8, 11].

Melanoma of the Nail Unit

Nail unit melanoma is a rare pathology corresponding to approximately 2–3% of all melanomas and usually occurs in advanced stages with an unfavorable prognosis. This melanoma is more prevalent in ethnic patients and its diagnosis is usual in ages between 50 and 70 years and rarely in pediatric patients. Unlike cutaneous malignant melanoma, nail melanoma is not related to sun exposure. It is believed that trauma, acute and chronic, plays an important role in the pathogenesis, since the majority of cases are located in the thumb or hallux, which are more exposed to trauma. Regarding its clinical presentation, it usually appears as a longitudinal melanonychia with a width greater than 3 mm and irregular borders in the nail plate. It is worth mentioning that 25–30% of nail unit melanomas can be amelanotic, presenting as longitudinal erythronychia or as a pink or red nodule. In addition, they may be accompanied by other signs such as onycholysis, fissures, bleeding or ulceration. This disease has may differential diagnosis, including benign etiologies. Although dermoscopy and onychoscopy are important clinical tools for recognizing patterns of malignancy, the do not have high sensitivity for the detection of all cases. Accordingly, biopsy of the nail matrix is considered the gold standard for diagnosis [2, 9, 12].

Diagnosis

Based in these photographs, clinical features, positive blood test, and the negative culture and KOH, the diagnosis of frictional subungual hematoma was done.

Discussion

Frictional subungual hematoma is caused by chronic repetitive microtrauma or friction that often goes unnoticed by the patient, who is usually asymptomatic. It is observed as a brownish-blackish dyschromia. In contrast, acute subungual hematoma, caused by an obvious blow, is accompanied by severe stabbing pain, edema and even active external bleeding. In the same way, frictional melanonychia is caused by the same injuries as frictional subungual hematoma, which cause damage to the nail matrix and consequently the activation of melanocytes, manifesting as a black-brown pigmentation, in the form of a longitudinal band, on the nail plate. These lesions, unlike skin hematomas, generally remains under the nail for a long time, since they are eliminated along with the growth of the nail. Therefore, a urine strip test of sub-nail material was performed to evaluate the presence of blood, which was positive. Furthermore, microscopy showed the presence of blood on the inner surface of the nail plate. These studies helped us to confirm the diagnosis. In the same way, subungual frictional pseudohematoma predominantly occurs in elderly patients with foot deformities, use of inappropriate footwear, and decreased dexterity in cleaning caring for toenails. It is important that when performing the physical examination of the nails, a correct cleaning and onychoscopic evaluation is carried out to rule out the presence of dirt under the nail and be able to reach an adequate diagnosis.

On the other hand, type 2 diabetes mellitus and advanced age are risk factors for onychomycosis. Fungal melanonychia is characterized by the presence of blackish pigmentation, produced by the deposit of melanin synthesized by the pathogen, associated with nail sings such as a hyperkeratosis and scales. Therefore, a culture and KOH of subungual tissue were requested, which both gave negative results.

It is essential to include melanoma of the nail unit as a differential diagnosis, since it represents a threat to the patient's life. This entity may present similar clinic features to the diagnoses described above, especially in the geriatric population. One of the most important pillars in the management of this pathology is the early diagnosis, an adequate clinical history, physical examination and histopathological evaluation are of utmost importance. In relation to the use of onychoscopy or dermoscopy, we must take into account the usefulness of the ABCDE rule of the Nail unit melanoma, for the recognition of clinical characteristics suggestive of malignancy. However, this tool is not sensitive enough, so taking a biopsy with its respective histopathological study continues to be the best detection method.

Key Points

For the diagnosis of subungual frictional hematoma, it is important to consider:

1. On physical examination, it is seen as a partial, total or longitudinal brown-black dyschromia with or without onycholysis. Onychoscopy shows the presence of a red-purple-brown pattern under the nail plate, homogeneous color and peripheral fading [2–6, 8, 9].
2. Investigate the use of shoes with steel or narrow toe, deformities of the toes, occupation and sports. Regarding location, they usually affect feet with predominancy in the first toes [1–4, 6, 7].
3. If there is doubt about the diagnosis, any methods of blood detection can be used, such as urine strip test or fecal occult blood test [4, 6, 7, 10].

References

1. Algoblan S, Turkumani MG, Altalhab S. Subungual hematoma treated successfully with 2940 nm erbium YAG Laser. Our Dermatol Online. 2018;9(2):218–9. https://doi.org/10.7241/ourd.20182.31.

2. Piraccini BM, Dika E, Fanti PA. Tips for diagnosis and treatment of nail pigmentation with practical algorithm. Dermatol Clin. 2015;33(2):185–95. https://doi.org/10.1016/j.det.2014.12.002.
3. Chang P, Haneke E, Borjas C, Pellecer D. Podal su ungual frictional haematoma. DCMQ. 2012;10(1):48–50. Available at: https://www.medigraphic.com/pdfs/cosmetica/dcm-2012/dcm121j.pdf
4. Chang P, Haneke E, Rodas A. Hematomas of the nail apparatus. DCMQ. 2009;7(3):196–201. Available at: https://www.medigraphic.com/pdfs/cosmetica/dcm-2009/dcm093h.pdf
5. Perper M, Tosti A. Chapter 6: Nail diseases in the elderly. In: Tosti A, editor. Nail disorders. 1st ed. Elsevier; 2019. p. 49–54. https://doi.org/10.1016/c2016-0-04563-1.
6. Chang P. Subungueal frictional hematoma due to overlaping toes. DCMQ. 2009;7(2):138–40. Available at: https://www.medigraphic.com/pdfs/cosmetica/dcm-2009/dcm092n.pdf
7. Chang P. Sunungual frictional pseudohematoma due to toe deformity. Aproposal of terminology and a report of 4 cases in elderly. DCMQ. 2009;7(3):160–3. Available at: https://www.medigraphic.com/pdfs/cosmetica/dcm-2009/dcm093b.pdf
8. Starace M, Alessandrini A, Brandi N, Piraccini BM. Use of nail dermoscopy in the management of melonychia: review. Dermatol Pract Concept. 2019;9(1):38–43. https://doi.org/10.5826/dpc.0901a10.
9. Tosti A, Piraccini BM, de Farias DC. Dealing with melanonychia. Semin Cutan Med Surg. 2009;28(1):49–54. https://doi.org/10.1016/j.sder.2008.12.004.
10. Huang Y-H, Ohara K. Medical pearl: subungual hematoma: a simple and quick method for diagnosis. J Am Acad Dermatol. 2006;54(5):877–8. https://doi.org/10.1016/j.jaad.2005.10.043.
11. Kim H-J, Kim T-W, Park S-M, et al. Clinical and dermoscopic features of fungal melanonychia: differentiating from subungual melanoma. Ann Dermatol. 2020;32(6):460. https://doi.org/10.5021/ad.2020.32.6.460.
12. Conway J, Bellet JS, Rubin AI, Lipner SR. Adult and pediatric nail unit melanoma: epidemiology, diagnosis, and treatment. Cells. 2023;12(6):964. https://doi.org/10.3390/cells12060964.

Chapter 8
Case Report: Onychomatricoma

Soumiya Chiheb ⓘ, Hanane Rachadi ⓘ, and Farida Marnissi

Abstract Onychomatricoma is a rare, benign tumor of the nail matrix that occurs in the middle age.

Clinically, and classicaly it presents with the tetrad of exaggerated transverse curvature, nail plate thickening, splinter hemorrhages, and leuco-xanthonychia.

Common dermoscopic features include longitudinal parallel white or yellow lines, parallel lesion edges, splinter hemorrhages, and the characteristic honeycomb-like cavities at the free edge.

Onychomatricoma is commonly misdiagnosed as onychomycosis.

The diagnosis is based on clinical and dermoscopic features like in our case Surgical excision remains the preferred treatment for onychomatricoma. After exposing the tumor by removing the nail plate and releasing the proximal fold, complete tangential excision is necessary to prevent recurrence.

After excision and on histological examination, the longitudinal sections of the onychomatricoma show a gloved, spindly finger appearance lined by matrical epithelium.

Here we describe a case of a 70-year-old man with onychomatricoma of his left ring finger.

The diagnosis suspected clinically was confirmed by the dermoscopy of the free edge with the aspect of honey comb-like cavities.

Keywords Onychomatricoma · Dermoscopy · Honey comb-like cavities

S. Chiheb (✉) · H. Rachadi
Faculty of Medicine and Pharmacy, Hassan II University, Department of Dermatology, Ibn Rochd University Hospital, Casablanca, Morocco

F. Marnissi
Faculty of Medicine and Pharmacy, Hassan II University, Department of Pathology, Ibn Rochd University Hospital, Casablanca, Morocco

Clinical Case

A 70-year-old man, retired and treated for glaucoma, presented with a color modification of the nail plate of his left ring finger, evolving for 3 years. A progressive thickening of the nail plate, which bled when cut, marked the progression. Clinically, we observed longitudinal leuko-xanthonychia with intercepted red and white-yellowish lines, filiform hemorrhage, disappearance of the lunar crescent, and pinkish background. The free edge of the nail plate revealed thickening and exaggerated transverse curvature (Fig. 8.1). The dermoscopic examination confirmed the clinical presentation by showing longitudinal parallel white and yellowish lines and splinter hemorrhage (Fig. 8.2a). The free edge dermoscopic examination showed thickening of the nail plate with honeycomb-like cavities (Fig. 8.2b). The histopathology showed a fibroepithelial villous tumor of the matrix with multiple 'glove finger' digitations along its connective tissue axes (Figs. 8.3a and 8.3b).

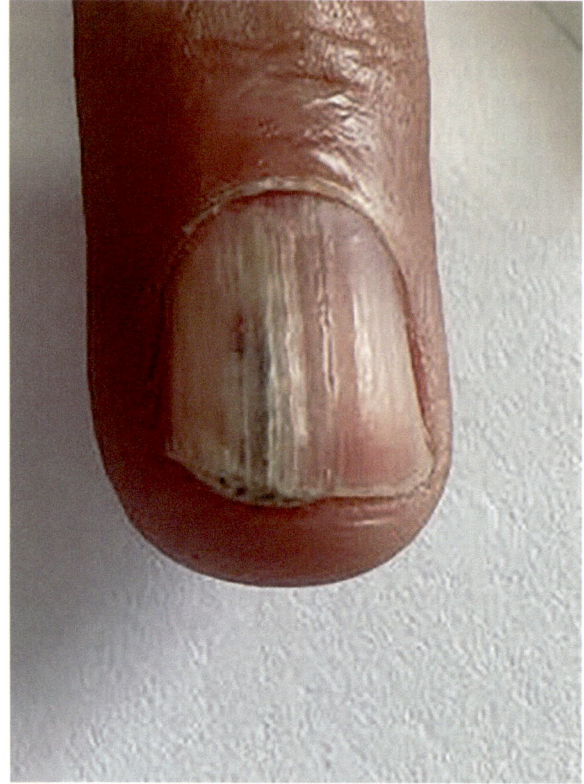

Fig. 8.1 longitudinal leuko-xanthonychia of a fingernail with filiform hemorrhage, the disappearance of the lunar crescent, and pinkish background

Fig. 8.2a Dermoscopy,
longitudinal parallel white
and yellowish lines and
splinter hemorrhage

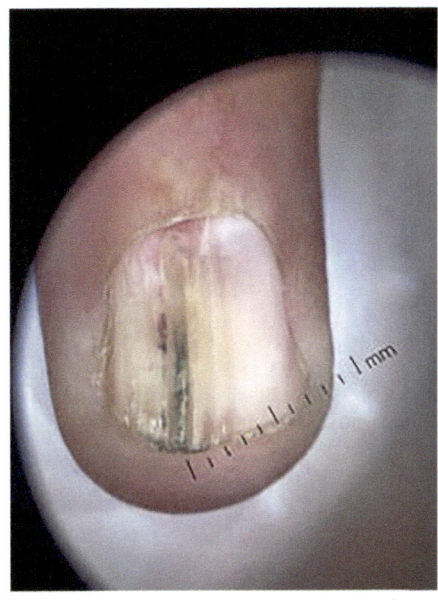

Fig. 8.2b Dermoscopy of
the free edge, honeycomb-
like cavities

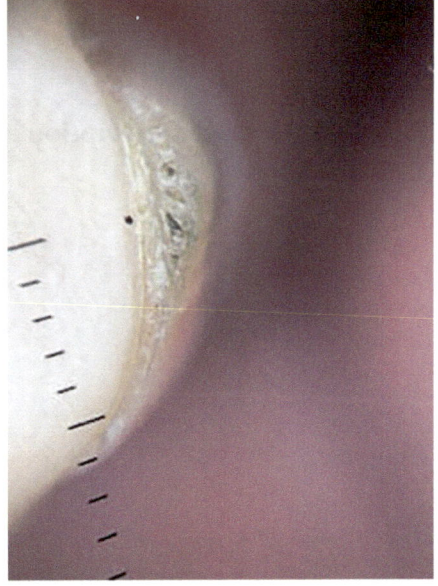

Fig. 8.3a Fibroepithelial
villous tumor of the matrix
with multiple 'glove
finger' digitations along its
connective tissue axes
(distal zone). (H&E, X10)

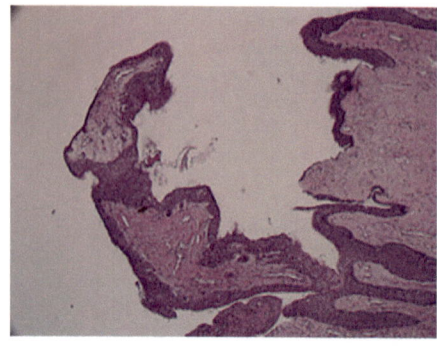

Fig. 8.3b Fibroepithelial
tumor with deep epithelial
invaginations. (H&E, X10)

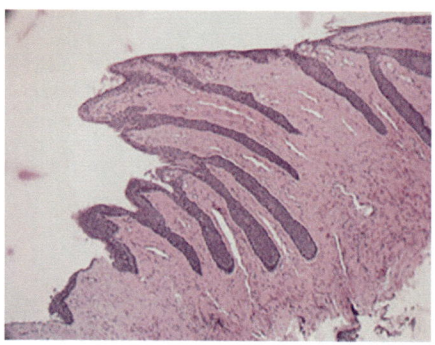

Based on the Case Description and the Photographs, What Is Your Diagnosis?

Onychomatricoma
Dermatophytoma
Nail psoriasis
Subungual wart

Diagnosis

Onychomatricoma

Discussion

Onychomatricoma is a rare, benign tumor of the nail matrix [1] with no more than 200 cases reported in the literature. It was first described in 1992 by Baran and Kint [2]. It can be diagnosed in individuals of both genders, ranging from 4 to 72 years old, but it predominantly occurs in middle-aged white women [1].

Classically, it presents as an asymptomatic slow-growing tumor with filamentous digitations originating from the nail matrix [3]. However, recent findings suggest that onychomatricoma can originate from areas of cell differentiation associated with the formation of matrix cells, which may be the ventral portion of the proximal nail fold [4] or the nail bed [5]. This tumor develops in one-third of cases at the fingernails [1]. The nails on the dominant hand are most frequently affected, particularly the thumb, and second and third fingers, while the great toe is the most commonly involved toenail [6]. Clinically, onychomatricoma presents with the tetrad of exaggerated transverse curvature, nail plate thickening, splinter hemorrhages, and leuco-xanthonychia [7] like in our case. Other nail findings may include longitudinal melanonychia, subungual hematoma, thickened proximal ungual fold, and dorsal pterygium [8]. Additionally, villous digitations emerging from the nail matrix are a characteristic intraoperative finding [9].

Dermoscopy proves highly beneficial in assessing suspected onychomatricoma cases, especially the dermoscopy of the free edge. Common dermoscopic features include longitudinal parallel white or yellow lines, parallel lesion edges, splinter hemorrhages, and the characteristic honeycomb-like cavities at the free edge [10].

Onychomatricoma is commonly misdiagnosed as onychomycosis. Other potential differential diagnoses include fibrokeratoma of the nail matrix, squamous cell carcinoma, Bowen's disease, viral warts, nail fibroma, and longitudinal melanonychia [1].

Imaging studies such as ultrasonography and magnetic resonance imaging can provide additional support for the diagnosis. The tumorous digit-like projections manifest as hyperechoic linear dots in ultrasonography and as a Y-shaped structure exhibiting high-intensity signals in magnetic resonance imaging [3]. These investigations are not mandatory in case of typical clinical and dermoscopic presentation. Direct surgical exploration is required, like in our case.

On histological examination, the longitudinal sections of the onychomatricoma show a gloved, spindly finger appearance lined by matrical epithelium. Proximally, transverse sections show a connective tissue tumor with a mamillated surface pierced by regular epithelial invaginations comprised of matrical epithelium. Distally, transverse sections show a nail plate that is markedly thickened with multiple empty cavities [6]. Nail clipping, which is a minimally invasive technique, can be used to confirm the diagnosis of onychomatricoma. Histological examination of the nail clipping reveals lacunae filled with serous fluid [7].

Surgical excision remains the preferred treatment for onychomatricoma. After exposing the tumor by removing the nail plate and releasing the proximal fold, complete tangential excision is necessary to prevent recurrence (Figs. 8.4a and 8.4b).

Key Points

When observing a painless, single-finger nail abnormality characterized by xanthonychia, transverse hypercurvature, filiform hemorrhage, dystrophy, and honeycomb-like cavities on dermoscopy of the nail plate's free edge,

Fig. 8.4a Intraoperative view of onychomatricoma after dissection of the proximal nail fold and excision of the nail plate

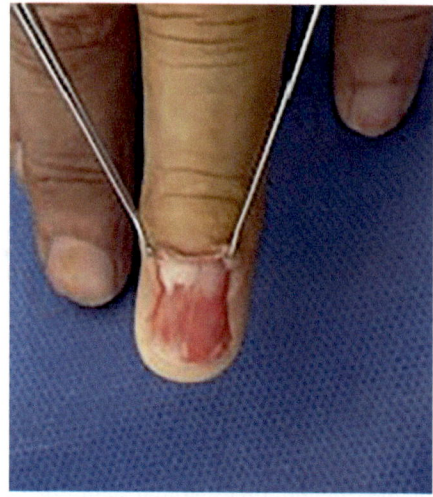

Fig. 8.4b Intraoperative view after resection of the tumor and repositioning of the proximal nail fold

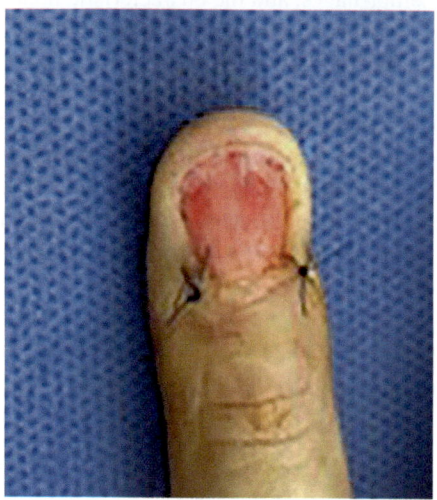

onychomatricoma should be considered. The management of this benign nail tumor is based on surgical exploration by a nail expert, this allows complete excision of the tumor and normal regrowth of the nail.

References

1. Di Chiacchio N, Tavares GT, Tosti A, et al. Onychomatricoma: epidemiological and clinical findings in a large series of 30 cases. Br J Dermatol. 2015;173(5):1305–7. https://doi.org/10.1111/bjd.13900.
2. Baran R, Kint A. Onychomatrixoma. Filamentous tufted tumor in the matrix of a funnel-shaped nail: a new entity (report of three cases). Br J Dermatol. 1992;126(5):510–5. https://doi.org/10.1111/j.1365-2133.1992.tb11827.x.
3. Jaeger TNG, Canella C, Leverone AP, Nakamura RC. Onychomatricoma with onychomycosis: a case report and review of the literature. Skin Appendage Disord. 2021;7(5):422–6. https://doi.org/10.1159/000516662.
4. Perrin C, Baran R. Onychomatricoma with dorsal pterygium: pathogenic mechanisms in 3 cases. J Am Acad Dermatol. 2008;59(6):990–4. https://doi.org/10.1016/j.jaad.2008.07.040.
5. Figueira B, de Mello CD, Noriega LF, Gioia Di Chiacchio N, Ocampo-Garza J, Di Chiacchio N. Onychomatricoma of the nail bed. Skin Appendage Disord. 2019;5(3):165–8. https://doi.org/10.1159/000494096.
6. Romero LS, Park H, Shoaee N, Cohen PR. Onychomatricoma presenting as a dystrophic right great toenail: case report and review. Cureus. 2020;12(5):e7946. https://doi.org/10.7759/cureus.7946.
7. Joshi TP, Dunn C, Huttenbach YT, Kim SJ. Onychomatricoma in a patient with skin of color. JAAD Case Rep. 2023;41:44–5. https://doi.org/10.1016/j.jdcr.2023.08.046.
8. Grover C, Gaurav V, Sharma S, Sinha S. Pigmented onychomatricoma presenting as pachymelanonychia striata: a case report and review of literature. Skin Appendage Disord. 2023;9(5):366–72. https://doi.org/10.1159/000529820.
9. Perrin C, Ambrosetti D. Pleomorphic onychomatricoma: a mimicker of malignancy. Acta Derm Venereol. 2022;102:adv00628. https://doi.org/10.2340/actadv.v101.546.
10. Lesort C, Debarbieux S, Duru G, Dalle S, Poulhalon N, Thomas L. Dermoscopic features of Onychomatricoma: a study of 34 cases. Dermatology. 2015;231(2):177–83. https://doi.org/10.1159/000431315.

Chapter 9
Red Lunulae Heralding Onychomadesis in Alopecia Areata

Tejashri Venkatesh, Victor L. Quan, Edward B. Li, Zachary J. Solomon, Andrea M. Rustad, and Maria L. Colavincenzo

Abstract In this case, development of red lunulae of all fingernails coincided with rapid onset of severe alopecia areata, which progressed to alopecia universalis with onychomadesis of all fingernails. Janus kinase inhibitor therapy improved the nail condition.

Keywords Alopecia areata · Nail abnormalities · Onychomadesis · Red lunulae · Janus kinase inhibitor

Clinical Case

A 41-year-old male with a history of moderate-severe atopic dermatitis since childhood and a 6-month history of biopsy-proven alopecia areata, presented with accelerated diffuse hair loss from the scalp, face and body, and new-onset discoloration of the fingernails (Figs. 9.1a and 9.1b). His medications at the time included minoxidil 5% foam and fluocinonide 0.05% solution to the scalp daily, as well as ketoconazole 2% shampoo every other day. He had once previously received intralesional triamcinolone injections to the scalp.

T. Venkatesh · V. L. Quan · E. B. Li · A. M. Rustad · M. L. Colavincenzo (✉)
Department of Dermatology, Northwestern University, Feinberg School of Medicine, Chicago, IL, USA

Chicago Medical School at Rosalind Franklin University, North Chicago, IL, USA
e-mail: tejashri.venkatesh@my.rfums.org; victor.quan@northwestern.edu; edward.li@nm.org; maria.colavincenzo@nm.org

Z. J. Solomon
Rush Copley Medical Center, Aurora, IL, USA

© The Author(s), under exclusive license to Springer Nature Switzerland AG 2025
A. Tosti et al. (eds.), *Clinical Cases in Nail Disorders*, Clinical Cases in Dermatology, https://doi.org/10.1007/978-3-031-88642-3_9

Four weeks later, the patient reported peeling up of all fingernails at the base (Fig. 9.2). His fingernails showed progressive trachyonychia, onycholysis and ultimately, onychomadesis over the following 6 weeks (Fig. 9.3). At this time, he was initiated on oral baricitinib 4 mg daily. The patient noted significant improvement in his fingernails after 3 months of treatment (Fig. 9.4). However, after 5 months of baricitinib therapy, his hair loss progressed to alopecia universalis, so the patient was switched to oral tofacitinib 5 mg twice daily. In the subsequent year on this regimen, his fingernails remained normal, although he did not experience any hair regrowth. He also noted a significant increase in atopic dermatitis disease activity during this time.

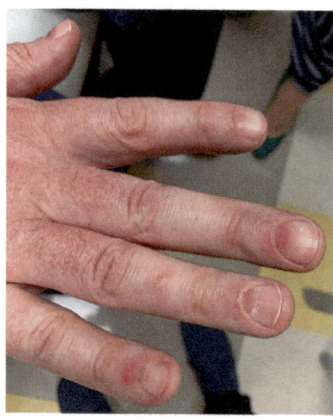

Fig. 9.1a Red lunulae on all five fingernails of the right hand. (Photo credits to co-author Solomon)

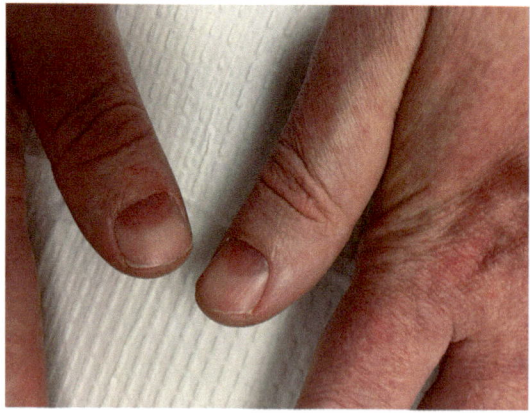

Fig. 9.1b Red lunulae on bilateral thumbs. (Photo credits to co-author Solomon)

Fig. 9.2 Trachyonychia of all five fingernails of the right hand. (Photo credits to the patient)

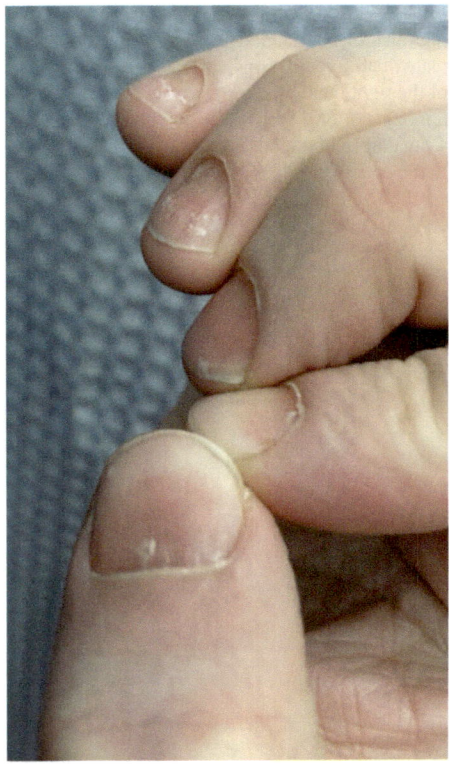

Fig. 9.3 Onychomadesis of all five fingernails of the right hand. (Photo credits to the patient)

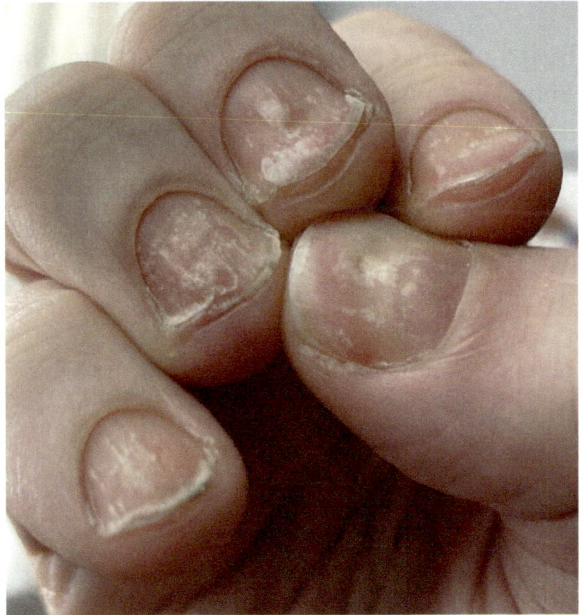

Fig. 9.4 Proximal
regrowth of normal nail
plate in all five fingernails
of the right hand after
3 months of oral baricitinib
4 mg daily. (Photo credits
to the patient)

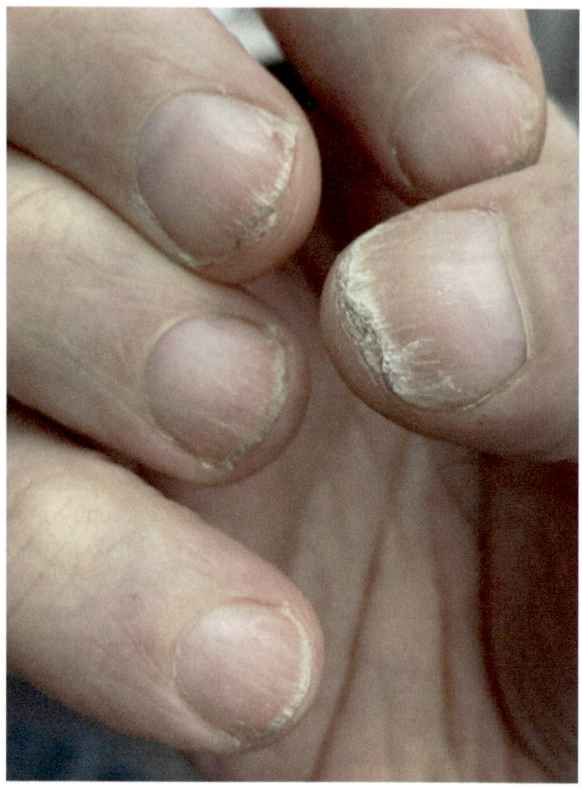

Based on the Case Description and the Photographs, What Is Your Diagnosis?

Alopecia areata-associated nail disease
Medication-induced nail changes
Psoriatic nail disease
Lichen planus
Hair and nail manifestations of lupus erythematosus

Diagnosis

Alopecia areata-associated nail disease

Discussion

Nail changes frequently occur in alopecia areata (AA) with an average prevalence of 30% and a wide spectrum of clinical manifestations [1]. Regular, geographic pitting and trachyonychia are the most commonly observed changes, with an average prevalence of 20% and 8%, respectively [1]. Other less common findings reported include red or spotted lunulae, punctate leukonychia, and onycholysis [1, 2]. Rare cases of onychomadesis have been reported in the pediatric population [3].

Red lunulae were first described in 1954 in patients with heart failure [4]. Several studies have found red spotted lunula to be specific for severe AA, although infrequently observed [5–8]. In addition to AA, red lunulae have been reported to occur with a range of diseases including connective tissue diseases such as lupus erythematosus, dermatomyositis, systemic sclerosis, rheumatoid arthritis, polymyositis, Sjogren's syndrome; other inflammatory dermatoses such as psoriasis, lichen planus, lichen sclerosus; and chikungunya and lymphogranuloma venereum infections [9–16].

The pathogenesis of red lunulae remains unclear. Proposed mechanisms include increased nail matrix angiogenesis due to local or systemic inflammation, distended vasculature and greater arteriolar blood flow, and changes in optical properties of the nail plate allowing for augmented visibility of normal underlying nail bed vasculature [9, 16]. Distinct histopathologic features of increased vascularity in the superficial nail matrix papillary dermis have been correlated with the red clinical appearance, supporting the hypothesis of angiogenesis as a contributing factor [6]. Trachyonychia in AA results from exocytosis and spongiosis of the nail matrix [1]. When severe, this inflammation leads to temporary, complete inhibition of nail plate production and onychomadesis with subsequent regrowth of a new nail plate [17].

The relationship between AA and associated nail changes similarly is not well understood. Both hair follicles and nail units are similar in structure and growth, possessing immune protection in the healthy state; thus, the concept of AA resulting from loss of immune privilege may extend to nail involvement [1, 18]. Onset of nail changes does not correlate with onset or severity of hair loss and may occur at any time during the course of AA [1]. However, nail changes are more common with increased severity of alopecia [1, 5, 7]. Conversely, patients with AA and nail changes are more than 8 times more likely to progress to AA universalis or totalis phenotypes [19]. These associations suggest that nail changes portend a poor prognosis of AA and may be an independent risk factor for treatment-resistant AA [1].

AA-associated nail changes are most commonly mild and asymptomatic, and may go unnoticed on examination [1, 5]. However, in more severe cases, the nail changes may cause pain, functional impairment, and cosmetic disfigurement [1]. Nail dermoscopy, performed dry or with ultrasound gel, may be helpful in detecting subtle changes [20].

Successful treatment of AA universalis and associated nail symptoms, occasionally with lunular involvement, has been reported with systemic Janus kinase inhibitors, namely tofacitinib and baricitinib, with minimal to no adverse effects [1, 21]. In our patient's case, treatment with baricitinib successfully resolved his nail changes; however, both baricitinib and tofacitinib failed to control his scalp alopecia areata and atopic dermatitis.

Key Points

1. Red lunulae and onychomadesis are less common nail manifestations reported to occur with alopecia areata.
2. The presence of red lunulae is associated with greater alopecia severity in alopecia areata.
3. Systemic Janus kinase inhibitors are a promising treatment for alopecia areata-associated nail disease.

References

1. Chelidze K, Lipner SR. Nail changes in alopecia areata: an update and review. Int J Dermatol. 2018;57(7):776–83. https://doi.org/10.1111/ijd.13866.
2. Bergner T, Donhauser G, Ruzicka T. Red lunulae in severe alopecia areata. Acta Derm Venereol. 1992;72(3):203–5.
3. Tosti A, Morelli R, Bardazzi F, Peluso AM. Prevalence of nail abnormalities in children with alopecia areata. Pediatr Dermatol. 1994;11(2):112–5. https://doi.org/10.1111/j.1525-1470.1994.tb00562.
4. Terry R. Red half-moons in cardiac failure. Lancet. 1954;267(6843):842–4. https://doi.org/10.1016/s0140-6736(54)91932-7.
5. Roest YBM, van Middendorp HT, Evers AWM, van de Kerkhof PCM, Pasch MC. Nail involvement in alopecia areata: a questionnaire-based survey on clinical signs, impact on quality of life and review of the literature. Acta Derm Venereol. 2018;98(2):212–7. https://doi.org/10.2340/00015555-2810.
6. Morrissey KA, Rubin AI. Histopathology of the red lunula: new histologic features and clinical correlations of a rare type of erythronychia. J Cutan Pathol. 2013;40(11):972–5. https://doi.org/10.1111/cup.12218.
7. Shakoei S, Seifi G, Ghanami F, et al. Clinical and demographic characteristics associated with nail involvement in alopecia areata: a cross-sectional study of 197 patients. Health Sci Rep. 2024;7(4):e2020. Published 2024 Apr 1. https://doi.org/10.1002/hsr2.2020.
8. Shelley WB. The spotted lunula. A neglected nail sign associated with alopecia areata. J Am Acad Dermatol. 1980;2(5):385–7. https://doi.org/10.1016/s0190-9622(80)80360-4.
9. Haneke E. Nail psoriasis: clinical features, pathogenesis, differential diagnoses, and management. Psoriasis (Auckl). 2017;7:51–63. Published 2017 Oct 16. https://doi.org/10.2147/PTT.S126281.
10. Żychowska M, Żychowska M. Nail changes in lichen planus: a single-center study. J Cutan Med Surg. 2021;25(3):281–5. https://doi.org/10.1177/1203475420982554.

11. Jorizzo JL, Gonzalez EB, Daniels JC. Red lunulae in a patient with rheumatoid arthritis. J Am Acad Dermatol. 1983;8(5):711–4. https://doi.org/10.1016/s0190-9622(83)70085-x.
12. Tunc SE, Ertam I, Pirildar T, Turk T, Ozturk M, Doganavsargil E. Nail changes in connective tissue diseases: do nail changes provide clues for the diagnosis? J Eur Acad Dermatol Venereol. 2007;21(4):497–503. https://doi.org/10.1111/j.1468-3083.2006.02012.x.
13. Cohen PR. Red lunulae: case report and literature review. J Am Acad Dermatol. 1992;26(2 Pt 2):292–4. https://doi.org/10.1016/0190-9622(92)70037-g.
14. Kumar R, Sharma MK, Jain SK, Yadav SK, Singhal AK. Cutaneous manifestations of chikungunya fever: observations from an outbreak at a tertiary care hospital in Southeast Rajasthan, India. Indian Dermatol Online J. 2017;8(5):336–42. https://doi.org/10.4103/idoj.IDOJ_429_16.
15. García-Patos V, Bartralot R, Ordi J, Baselga E, de Moragas JM, Castells A. Systemic lupus erythematosus presenting with red lunulae. J Am Acad Dermatol. 1997;36(5 Pt 2):834–6. https://doi.org/10.1016/s0190-9622(97)70034-3.
16. Wilkerson MG, Wilkin JK. Red lunulae revisited: a clinical and histopathologic examination. J Am Acad Dermatol. 1989;20(3):453–7. https://doi.org/10.1016/s0190-9622(89)70057-8.
17. Braswell MA, Daniel CR 3rd, Brodell RT. Beau lines, onychomadesis, and retronychia: a unifying hypothesis. J Am Acad Dermatol. 2015;73(5):849–55. https://doi.org/10.1016/j.jaad.2015.08.003.
18. Kasumagic-Halilovic E, Prohic A. Nail changes in alopecia areata: frequency and clinical presentation. J Eur Acad Dermatol Venereol. 2009;23(2):240–1. https://doi.org/10.1111/j.1468-3083.2008.02830.x.
19. García-Hernández MJ, Rodríguez-Pichardo A. Multivariate analysis in alopecia areata: risk factors and validity of clinical forms. Arch Dermatol. 1999;135(8):998–9. https://doi.org/10.1001/archderm.135.8.998.
20. Haenssle HA, Blum A, Hofmann-Wellenhof R, et al. When all you have is a dermatoscope-start looking at the nails. Dermatol Pract Concept. 2014;4(4):11–20. https://doi.org/10.5826/dpc.0404a02. Published 2014 Oct 31
21. Rózsa P, Degovics D, Baltás E, Gyulai R, Kemény L. Successful treatment of alopecia areata-associated trachyonychia with baricitinib. Int J Dermatol. 2024;63:1089–90. https://doi.org/10.1111/ijd.17137. Published online March 21, 2024

Chapter 10
A 6-Year-Old Girl with Oyster Shell-Like Toenails

Katerina Damevska ⓘ **and Ordanche Ribarski**

Abstract A 6-year-old girl is referred for an appointment at the University Clinic for Dermatology in Skopje due to her laterally deviated, thickened, yellowish-brown discolored toenails with grooves. The toenail changes began at the age of one, followed by two episodes of nail plate detachment and regrowth of identical toenail plates. Based on a suspected fungal infection, the patient underwent treatment with oral and topical antifungals. Despite the antifungal treatment, no signs of improvement were observed.

Based on the clinical presentation, five differential diagnoses came into consideration: physiological nail alterations, pachyonychia congenita, yellow nail syndrome, retronychia, and congenital malalignment of the great toenails (CMGT). Out of the established differential diagnoses, the CMGT matches at most with the clinical presentation of our patient. As in Samman's description toenails appear yellowish-brown, discolored, oyster-shell-like shaped with a lateral deviation from mild ($<10^0$), moderate (10–20^0), to severe ($>20^0$). This lateral deviation can further lead to onychogryphosis, onychomadesis, onychomycosis, retronychia, paronychia, or onycholysis which happened twice to our patient. Most cases of CMGT remain overlooked or are misdiagnosed in up to 85% as onychomycosis. In some patients, CMGT can resolve by itself, while in those with severe deviation, a surgical avulsion can be proposed.

Keywords Physiological nail alterations · Pachyonychia congenita · Yellow nail syndrome · Retronychia · Congenital Malalignment of the Great Toenails

K. Damevska (✉) · O. Ribarski
University Clinic for Dermatology, Faculty of Medicine, Ss Cyril and Methodius University in Skopje, Skopje, Macedonia

© The Author(s), under exclusive license to Springer Nature Switzerland AG 2025
A. Tosti et al. (eds.), *Clinical Cases in Nail Disorders*, Clinical Cases in Dermatology, https://doi.org/10.1007/978-3-031-88642-3_10

A 6-year-old, healthy girl presented with a history of yellowish-brown-colored and thickened toenails since one year old. Due to the thickening, the girls' mother noted that the nails cannot be trimmed with a nail clipper. Occasionally, the girl complained of pain when walking and running. At 2–3 years old, both toenail plates detached from the nail bed, followed by regrowth of nail plates with identical changes. Nail specimens were collected many times due to a suspected fungal infection. Repeated mycological cultures showed either a negative result or the presence of yeast. Despite the prescribed course of oral antifungal medication and persistent use of topical antifungals, no signs of improvement were observed. At last, surgical avulsion of both toenails was advised, but the girls' mother refused it.

The physical examination revealed lateral deviation of the great toenail, discoloration, and oyster shell-like thickened nail plate with grooves of both toenails (Figs. 10.1 and 10.2). Inflammation of nail folds was not observed. Direct microscopic examination was negative.

Fig. 10.1 Clinical appearance of the patients' great toenails. Green-brown discoloration of the right great toenail with grooves and trapezoid shape on the free end of the nail plate. Slower growth rate and shortening of the nail plate of the left great toenail

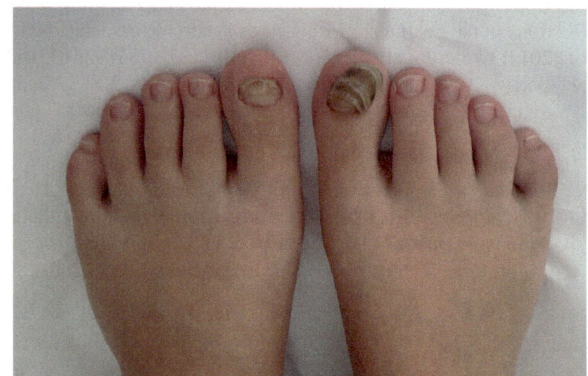

Fig. 10.2 "Oyster shell" appearance: multiple transverse grooves across the nail

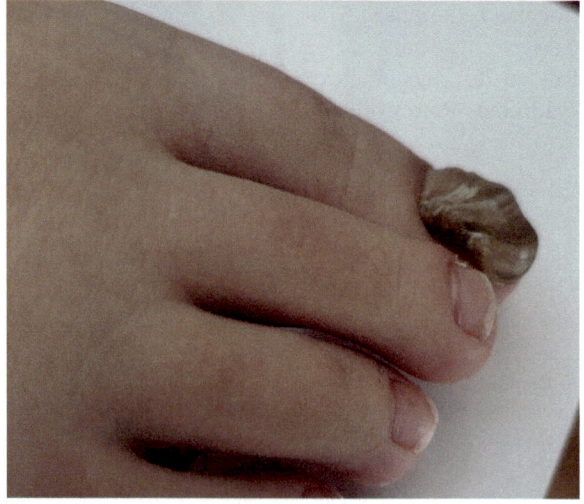

Based on the Case Description and the Photographs, What Is Your Diagnosis?

1. Physiological nail alterations
2. Pachyonychia congenita
3. Yellow nail syndrome
4. Retronychia
5. Congenital Malalignment of the Great Toenails

Diagnosis

Congenital Malalignment of the Great Toenails

Discussion

Nail changes are rare among the pediatric population and are often not brought to the attention of physicians; thus, they are overlooked.

The nail changes might represent typical age-related nail alterations or abnormalities that require medical attention. Often, thin, soft, and miniature nail plates add to the difficulty of making the correct diagnosis. The incidence varies from 3% to 11% and is influenced by socioeconomic and environmental factors [1]. Since nail disorders often go undetected, the number of affected children significantly exceeds the actual number of diagnosed patients.

[2]. Physiological alterations that do not require treatment and typically fade away with aging. A detailed review of physiological alterations of nail plates in pediatric patients is presented in Table 10.1.

Nail disorders in children are broadly categorized into congenital and acquired diseases.

Pachyonychia congenita is a rare, autosomal dominantly inherited genodermatosis caused by a mutation in one of the keratin genes (*KRT6A, KRT6B, KRT6C, KRT16,* and *KRT17*) [1, 2]. The disease's primary characteristics are hyperkeratotic, yellowish-brown toenail plates with a heightened curvature and difficulty to trim [2, 3, 5]. However, the association of nail changes with palmoplantar keratoderma, follicular hyperkeratosis, and benign oral leukokeratosis makes this diagnosis less likely [1].

Yellow nail syndrome [OMIM 153300] rarely affects pediatric patients. On the contrary, this rare disease usually affects the elderly over the age of 50 without sex predominance. The prevalence is estimated to be 1:100,000. A combination of nail changes, respiratory pathology, and lymphedema makes up the pathognomonic triad of the yellow nail syndrome. The nails appear yellow (xanthonychia),

Table 10.1 Overview of the physiological alterations of nails in children [1, 3, 4]

Physiological alteration	Definition	Affected age group	Etiology
Pseudo-Ingrown toenail	Pseudohypertrophy of the toenail's proximal and lateral folds without signs of inflammation	Newborns	Overlap of the toenail's folds as the thin, triangular-shaped nail plate pushes them down
Koilonychia	Nail plates with a transversal and longitudinal concavity are called "spoon-shaped" nails.	Newborns	Hereditary, acquired (iron-deficiency anemia related) or idiopathic
Onychoschizia	Brittle nails with a transverse, lamellar splitting at the free margin of the nail plate, usually on the big toes or thumbs	Newborns	Repeated bathing, watering or nail-sucking
Beau's lines	Solitary transverse nail groove presented usually at the age of 4 weeks	Infancy (1 month to 1 year)	Intrauterine distress, labor-related trauma, or mild trauma on the proximal nail matrix
Punctate leukonychia	Milky white colored foci due to the presence of parakeratotic cells within the nail plate	Toddlers (1–3 years)	Ill-fitting shoe trauma transmitted to the distal nail matrix causes abnormal keratinization.
Chevron nails	Oblique, longitudinal ridges converge towards the center of the nail plate's free margin.	Preschoolers (3–5 years)	The etiology remains unclear

hardened (scleronychia), and curved; likewise, our patient [6]. However, respiratory disease or lymphedema must be present to conclude the diagnosis. Bilateral exudative pleural effusions with lymphocytic cell predominance, bronchiectasis, chronic cough, recurrent pneumonia, and sinusitis are yellow-nail syndrome patients' most common pulmonary findings [6, 7]. Another distinctive clinical feature is lymphedema, which affects the lower extremities in 30 to 80% of the patients [6]. Due to the clinical presentation, yellow nail syndrome is unlikely to be the correct diagnosis.

Retronychia is a pattern of nail ingrowth first described by De Berker and Rendall1 in 1999. The combination of nail plate ingrowth into the proximal nail fold is associated with multiple generations of nail plate misaligned beneath the proximal nail, persistent inflammation (paronychia), and granulation tissue formation. The disease's onset usually follows either a prior footwear trauma or a systemic disease with a subsequent proximal nail plate detachment from the underlying matrix [8]. Management of retronychia consists of complete avulsion of the nail plate.

Onychomadesis is considered an extreme form of Beau line with subsequent separation of the proximal nail plate from the nail bed. Both fall along a spectrum of nail plate abnormalities secondary to temporary nail matrix arrest [9]. Various disorders have been reported in association with onychomadesis, including autoimmune and inflammatory diseases (alopecia areata, pemphigus vulgaris, vasculitis, bullous pemphigoid), infectious diseases (hand-foot-mouth disease), and medication use (antiepileptic drugs, azithromycin, chemotherapeutics, lithium, penicillin V, and retinoid) and underwent trauma [9, 10]. Any etiological event can temporarily disturb the proliferative activity of the nail matrix and cause complete inhibition of nail plate production. When the nail matrix reestablishes proliferative activity, the new nail plate undermines the preexisting, discontinuous nail plate to the point where it sheds off [10]. To our knowledge, the patient did not experience any etiological events relevant to onychomadesis. Additionally, the yellowish, oyster shell-like nails with multiple Beau's lines do not match the clinical aspects of onychomadesis.

Out of the proposed differential diagnoses, the congenital malalignment of the great toenails most closely matches the clinical presentation of our 6-year-old patient.

Congenital malalignment of the great toenail (CMGT), also known as congenital malalignment syndrome, is an idiopathic deviation of the nail apparatus. Initially described by Samman in the 1970s, the disease often goes undiagnosed or misdiagnosed as onychomycosis in up to 85% of cases. Moreover, the antifungal drugs are ineffective and show no signs of improvement in cases of congenital malalignment of great toenails, just like in our patient [11, 12]. The "congenital" feature implies the possible autosomal dominant inheritance and the early onset of symptoms when the child starts to crawl and walk [12]. In the case of the 6-year-old girl, symptoms began when she turned 1 year old.

Nowadays, two proposed theories do not fully explain the clinical presentation of congenital malalignment of the great toenails. According to the first theory, the lateral nail plate deviation follows an abnormality in the connective ligament between the matrix and the periosteum of the distal phalange. The second theory is based on excessive nail plate traction secondary to the big toe's hypertrophic extensor tendon [11]. The lateral deviation varies from mild ($<10^0$), moderate ($10–20^0$), to severe ($>20^0$). The treatment can be either a conservative or surgical avulsion, depending on the severity of the lateral deviation [11]. As in Samman's description, the disease usually appears as bilaterally thickened, discolored, oyster shell-like nail plates with a lateral deviation apart from the long axis of the big toes. This deviation may further lead to discoloration (ranging from brownish-black to green-brown and yellow), onychogryphosis, onychomadesis, onychomycosis, onycholysis, paronychia, and retronychia [11, 12]. In the mother's words, onycholysis occurred twice, followed by the regrowth of identical toenails.

More recently, Buttars et al. reviewed all published cases of CMGT to assess its association with underlying lateral displacement of the distal phalange and disappearing nail bed (DNB) [12].

A correct diagnosis is required to prevent unnecessary treatments. The differential diagnosis includes onychomycosis, connective tissue disorders, nail apparatus tumors, and dermatoses with nail involvement. In some cases, CMGT may spontaneously resolve.

Surgical treatment may be considered in patients with severe forms until up to 2 years of age.

Key Points

- Nail disorders present differently in children than in adults. Physiological nail alterations in children must be distinguished from nail disorders since no treatment is required.
- Congenital malalignment of the great toenails (CMGT) may be observed in 1–2% of children.
- CMGT is rarely diagnosed, and in most cases, patients have been inadequately treated with oral and topical antifungals.
- Thickened, yellowish-colored, oyster shell-like toenail plates with an early onset and difficulty trimming can imply CMGT as a suspect diagnosis.
- Familiarity with CMGT is essential to reach an accurate diagnosis and provide better care.

Consent for Publication   Consent has been obtained to publish clinical data and imaging for this case report.

Conflict of Interest   The authors have no conflicts of interest to declare.

References

1. Starace M, Alessandrini A, Piraccini BM. Nail disorders in children. Skin Appendage Disord. 2018 Oct;4(4):217–29.
2. Piraccini BM, Starace M. Nail disorders in infants and children. Curr Opin Pediatr. 2014 Aug;26(4):440–5.
3. Richert B, André J. Nail disorders in children: diagnosis and management. Am J Clin Dermatol. 2011;12(2):101–12.
4. Singal A, Bisherwal K. Disorders of nail in infants and children. Indian J Paediatr Dermatol. 2019;20:101–11.
5. Wulkan AJ, Tosti A. Pediatric nail conditions. Clin Dermatol. 2013;31(5):564–72.
6. Cheslock M, Harrington DW. Yellow Nail Syndrome. [Updated 2022 Sept 19]. In: StatPearls [Internet]. Treasure Island (FL): StatPearls Publishing; 2024. Available from: https://www.ncbi.nlm.nih.gov/books/NBK557760/.
7. Vignes S, Baran R. Yellow nail syndrome: a review. Orphanet J Rare Dis. 2017;12(1):42.
8. de Berker DA, Richert B, Duhard E, Piraccini BM, André J, Baran R. Retronychia: proximal ingrowing of the nail plate. J Am Acad Dermatol. 2008;58(6):978–83.
9. Damevska K, Gocev G, Pollozahani N, Nikolovska S, Neloska L. Onychomadesis following cutaneous vasculitis. Acta Dermatovenerol Croat. 2017;25(1):77–9.
10. Hardin J, Haber RM. Onychomadesis: literature review. Br J Dermatol. 2015;172(3):592–6.
11. Domínguez-Cherit J, Lima-Galindo AA. Congenital malalignment of the great toenail: conservative and definitive treatment. Pediatr Dermatol. 2021;38(3):555–60.
12. Buttars B, Scott SG, Glinka D, Daniel CR, Brodell RT, Braswell MA. Congenital malalignment of the great toenail, the disappearing nail bed, and distal phalanx deviation: a review. Skin Appendage Disord. 2022;8(1):8–12.

Chapter 11
Periungual Chromoblastomycosis Successfully Treated with 5% Topical Imiquimod

Nilton Gioia Di Chiacchio (iD) **and Nilton Di Chiacchio** (iD)

Abstract The treatment of chromoblastomycosis is still not defined, without a well-established standard treatment. It is associated with low cure and high recurrence rates, leading to long treatment. Therapy options depend on the extent of the lesions, location and patient's comorbidities. We report an unusual case of chromoblastomycosis (*Fonsecaea pedrosoi*) treated exclusively with topical 5% imiquimod (5times/week for 9 months), followed by complete involution of the clinical lesions, and no recurrence after 4 years of follow-up.

Keywords Fonsecaea pedrosoi · Chromoblastomycosis · Imiquimod · Nail changes

Clinical Case

A 46-year-old man, Fitzpatrik III, presenting a periungual (third right finger—proximal nail fold) erythematous verrucous/keratotic nodule for 1 year (Fig. 11.1). Right limb was also affected by the same pattern of lesions (nodules and granulomatous plaques) (Fig. 11.2). Some of the lesions presented a scarring center. Onychoscopy allowed a better visualization of the keratotic surface of the periungual papule, with black-violaceous dots, corresponding to hemorrhages spots (Fig. 11.3). Histological examination of the periungual lesion

N. G. Di Chiacchio (✉)
Faculdade de Medicina do ABC, Santo André, SP, Brazil

Hospital do Servidor Público Municipal de São Paulo, Santo André, SP, Brazil

N. Di Chiacchio
Hospital do Servidor Público Municipal de São Paulo, Santo André, SP, Brazil

© The Author(s), under exclusive license to Springer Nature
Switzerland AG 2025
A. Tosti et al. (eds.), *Clinical Cases in Nail Disorders*, Clinical Cases in
Dermatology, https://doi.org/10.1007/978-3-031-88642-3_11

67

revealed pseudoepitheliomatous hyperplasia with absent granulosa layer and partially stratum corneum replaced by parakeratosis. In the superficial dermis, the presence of grouped brownish fungal spores is observed, distributed among neutrophilic leukocytes or also phagocytosed by multinucleated giant cells (Fig. 11.4).

Fig. 11.1 Erythematous verrucous nodule affecting the proximal nail fold of the third right finger

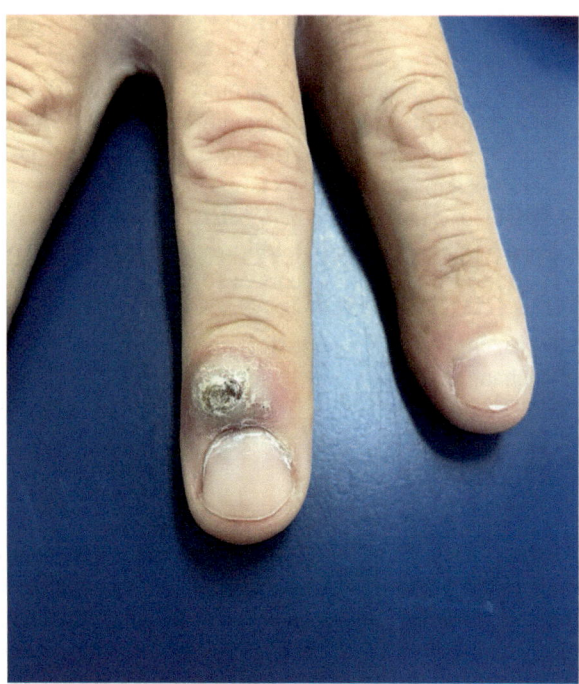

Fig. 11.2 Tumors and nodules were also presented in the right limb

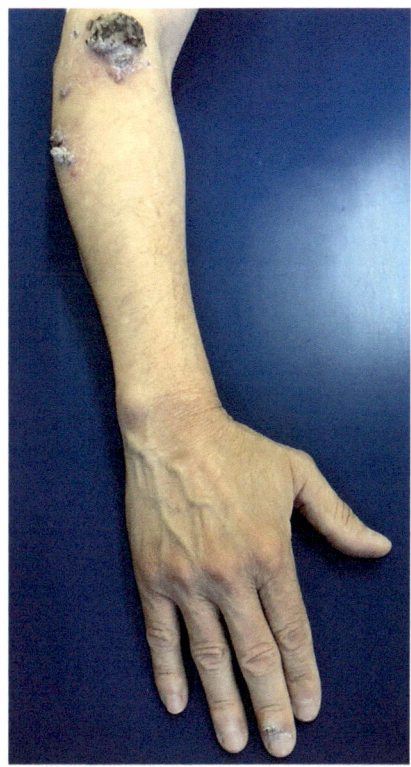

Fig. 11.3 Keratotic surface of the periungual papule, with black-violaceous dots

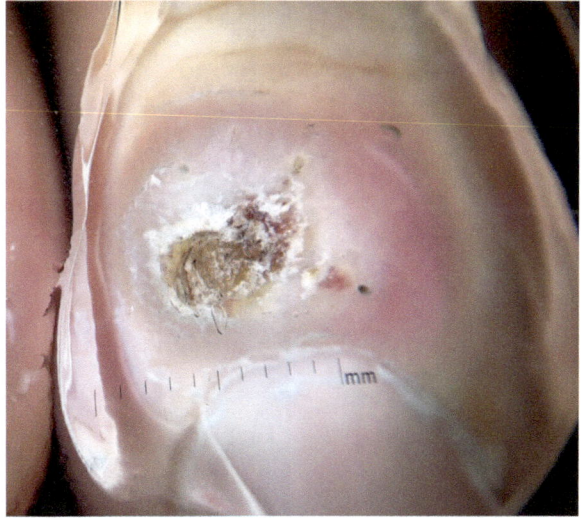

Fig. 11.4 Presence of grouped brownish fungal spores

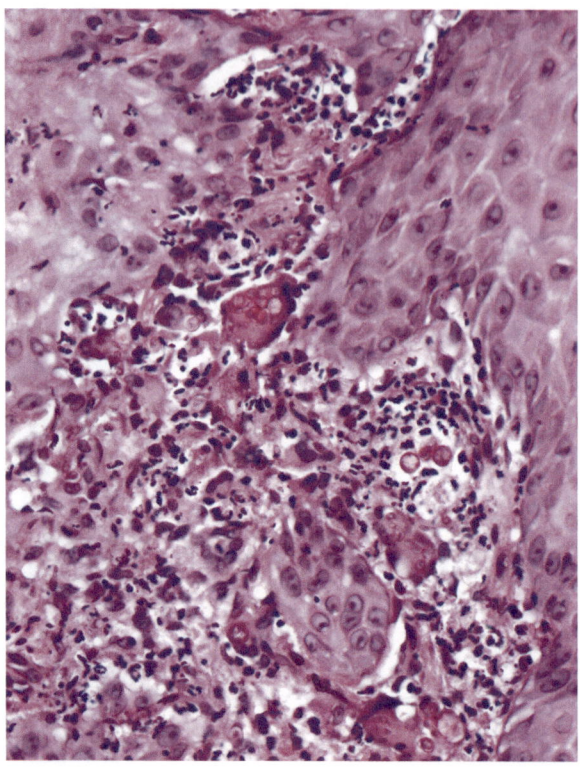

Fig. 11.5 Clinical aspect after 1 year of the use of topical 5% imiquimod

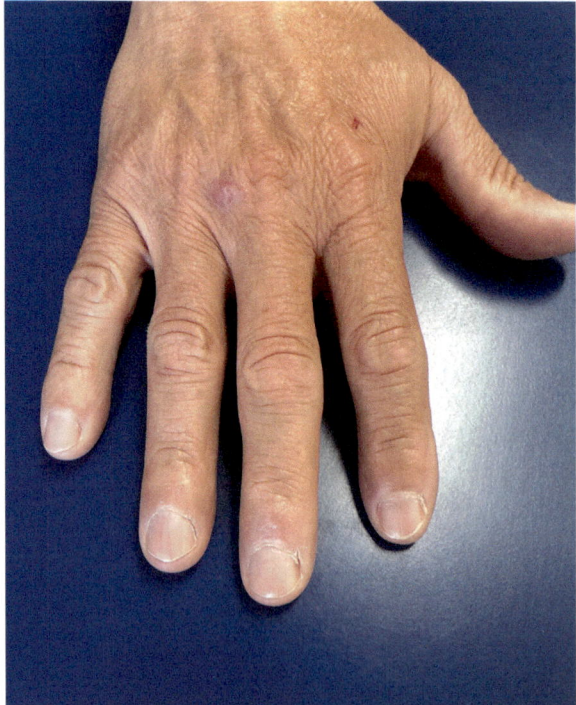

Based on the Case Description and the Photographs, What Is Your Diagnosis?

A. Cutaneous tuberculosis.
B. Syphilis.
C. Chromoblastomycosis.
D. Leishmaniasis.
E. Sporotrychosis.

Diagnosis

F. Chromoblastomycosis.

Discussion

Chromoblastomycosis is a chronic infectious dermatosis, classified as a subcutaneous implantation mycosis [1]. It is caused by the traumatic inoculation of dematiaceous fungi, with *Fonsecaea pedrosoi* being the most frequently isolated in Latin America [2, 3]. Clinically, it presents in a polymorphic, oligosymptomatic form, and may take months to develop. The most prevalent clinical expression is the verrucous form, which can spread contiguously, lymphatic or hematogenously [1]. It particularly affects the lower limbs, with only one case described of nail involvement [4].

We report an unusual case of chromoblastomycosis (*Fonsecaea pedrosoi*) treated exclusively with topical 5% imiquimod (5 times/week for 9 months), followed by complete involution of the clinical lesions (Fig. 11.5). The patient did not receive any other type of treatment (topical and/or systemic), before or after the use of topical imiquimod. Cure was confirmed by histopathology, after 1 year of the clinical cure. No recurrence was observed after 4 years of follow-up.

The treatment of chromoblastomycosis is still not defined, without a well-established standard treatment. It is associated with low cure and high recurrence rates, leading to long treatment. Therapy options depend on the extent of the lesions, location and patient's comorbidities [1]. Many treatments are described, including systemic therapy with oral and intravenous antifungals (itraconazole/terbinafine/amphotericin B/5-fluorocytosine), surgical excision and physical therapies (cryotherapy and thermotherapy).

Recently, the use of topical immunomodulators, such as imiquimod, has been described as potential therapeutic agents for non-infectious, and infectious diseases, such as chromoblastomycosis [5–7].

The successful treatment demonstrated in this case, as well as in other cases published, corroborates the action of imiquimod as a modulator of the anti-fungal response and an effective and promising therapy for chromoblastomycosis. However, new studies with a larger number of patients are needed to confirm the effectiveness of this treatment.

Key Points

Nail chromoblastomycosis is rare.

The classic treatment of chromoblastomycosis, based on itraconazole and/or terbinafine as well as physical approaches, is considered complex and ineffective due to the high relapses rate.

Topical imiquimod has been successfully described as potential therapeutic agents for chromoblastomycosis.

References

1. Brito AC, Bittencourt MJS. Chromoblastomycosis: an etiological, epidemiological, clinical, diagnostic and treatment up-date. An Bras Dermatol. 2018;93(4):495–506.
2. Queiroz-Telles F, et al. Mycoses of implantation in Latin America: an overview of epidemiology, clinical manifestations, diagnosis and treatment. Med Mycol. 2011;49(3):225–36.
3. Queiroz-Telles F, de Hoog S, Santos DWCL, Salgado CG, Vicente VA, Bonifaz A, Roilides E, Xi L, Azevedo CDMPES, da Silva MB, Pana ZD, Colombo AL, Walsh TJ. Chromoblastomycosis. Clin Microbiol Rev. 2017;30:233–76.
4. Sarti HM, et al. Longitudinal melanonychia secondary to chromoblastomycosis due to *Fonsecaea pedrosoi*. Int J Dermatol. 2008;47(7):764–5.
5. de Sousa M d GT, et al. Topical application of imiquimod as a treatment for chromoblastomycosis. Clin Infect Dis. 2014;58(12):1734–7.
6. da Glória Sousa M, et al. Restoration of pattern recognition receptor costimulation to treat chromoblastomycosis, a chronic fungal infection of the skin. Cell Host Microbe. 2011;9(5):436–43.
7. Belda W Jr, Criado PR, Passero LFD. Successful treatment of chromoblastomycosis caused by *Fonsecaea pedrosoi* using imiquimod. J Dermatol. 2020;47(4):409–12.

Chapter 12
A Painful Subungual Bluish Discoloration

Chander Grover (iD)

Abstract A 38-year-old female patient with bluish discoloration of left middle fin-gernail is presented. She complained of intense pain in this distinctive blue to purple discoloured area. Pin-point tenderness and onychoscopic changes suggested a nail bed glomus tumor. High frequency ultrasound revealed a 5.8 × 3.9 cm hypoechoic lesion on the radial aspect with increased vascularity. Magnetic resonance T1-weighted images showed an isointense lesion with intense contrast enhance-ment. A diagnosis of glomus tumor was confirmed and surgical excision was offered. A transungual excision, after proximal partial nail avulsion revealed a well-defined tumour (6 × 4 mm) with an irregular surface. Primary closure of the nail bed defect with nail plate repositioning was done. Histopathology of the excised speci-men confirmed the diagnosis. An uneventful post-operative recovery with no resid-ual pain, discoloration, or onycholysis was seen. The case is reported to outline the diagnostic and therapeutic approach and discuss possible differential diagnoses.

Keywords Glomus tumor · Subungual · Transungual · High-frequency ultrasound · Onychoscopy

Introduction

A blue discoloration of the nail can occur due to various etiologies. It is most com-monly due to a subungual hematoma; however, other causes include argyria (azure lunulae), chloronychia (occasionally blue), nail lichen planus (occasionally blue), hereditary acrolabial telangiectasia, nail bed cyanosis, Wilson's disease or drugs (commonly minocycline) [1–4]. A painful blue discoloration needs thorough evaluation. Although it may suggest a subungual hematoma, a nail tumor (espe-cially a vascular tumor) should also be suspected. This chapter discusses a

C. Grover (✉)
Department of Dermatology and STD, University College of Medical Sciences and GTB Hospital, Dilshad Garden, Delhi, India

© The Author(s), under exclusive license to Springer Nature Switzerland AG 2025
A. Tosti et al. (eds.), *Clinical Cases in Nail Disorders*, Clinical Cases in Dermatology, https://doi.org/10.1007/978-3-031-88642-3_12

73

38 year-old-woman who presented with a localised bluish discoloration of nail slowly increasing in size.

Case Details

A 38-year-old female patient presented to our outpatient department with bluish discoloration of her left middle fingernail, noticed for the past 12 months. It had initially started as a small area, but had progressively increased in size. The initial tenderness and discomfort had slowly worsened with occasional episodes of intense pain in the area. On examination, there was a distinctive area of blue to purple discoloration (Fig. 12.1). It was exquisitely painful on palpation. Pin-point tenderness (Love's pin test) was present. There were no nail fold or distal nail bed changes. Overlying nail plate was normal in appearance.

Onychoscopy revealed a normal nail plate without any surface abnormalities or areas of leukonychia. Nail bed showed a large, Ill-defined, bluish structureless area interspersed with reddish areas (especially distally) and a whitish zone (proximally) (Fig. 12.2). It was homogenous, with no evidence of globules, streaks or peripheral fading. There were no longitudinal bands of erythronychia, or visualised vessels. Though the lunula was not visualised, proximally there was a whitish area as described. There were no nail fold changes or capillary rarefaction in the proximal nail fold.

Fig. 12.1 Left middle fingernail showing a proximally placed area of bluish discoloration

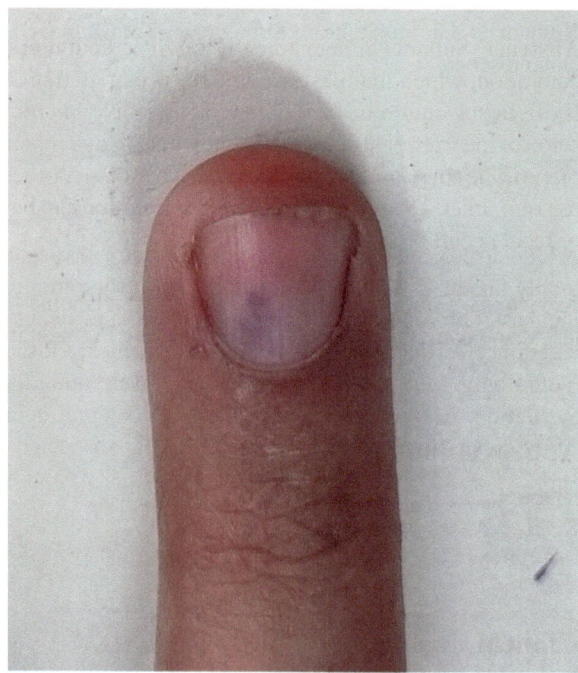

Fig. **12.2** Onychoscopy showing an ill-defined, homogenous, bluish structureless area in the left proximal nail bed. Distally there are interspersed reddish areas and proximally a whitish zone [10X Poarized]

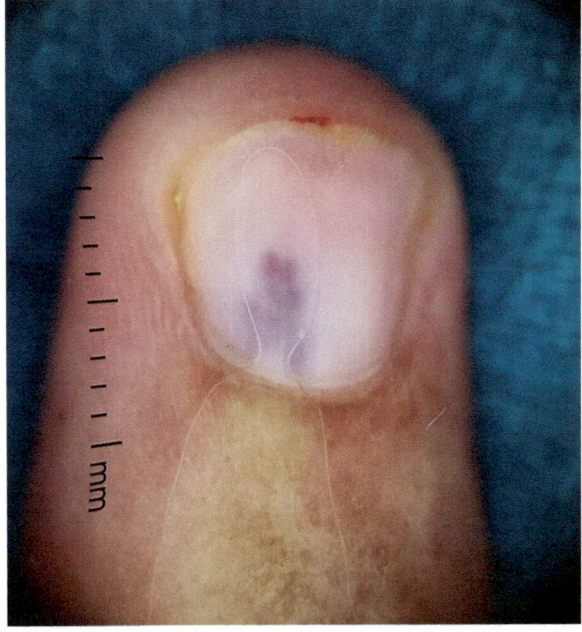

An ultrasound examination showed a 5.8 × 3.9 cm hypoechoic lesion, involving the nail bed, on the radial aspect, with an increased vascularity. It was extending towards the nail matrix. Magnetic resonance T1-weighted images showed an isointense lesion on the dorsal aspect of terminal phalanx of third finger with intense contrast enhancement. These findings were suggestive of a glomus tumor.

The patient was counselled regarding the need for surgical removal. After obtaining a written informed consent, digital anesthesia was administered in the form of proximal block. Exsanguination was done followed by tourniquet. Proximal partial nail avulsion was done to explore the area of bluish discoloration (Fig. 12.3a). The proximal nail fold was separated from bilateral lateral nail folds with full thickness radial incisions. It was retracted and held back with stay sutures. A well-defined tumour mass was seen involving the nail bed area, measuring 6 × 4 mm approximately. It had an irregular surface impinging on the distal nail matrix (Fig. 12.3b). The tumour was completely excised as a jelly like mass (Fig. 12.3c). The resultant defect (Fig. 12.3d) was carefully explored to look for any remnants. Intraoperative onychoscopy was done to ensure complete excision (Fig. 12.4). The nail bed defect was closed with 5–0 absorbable suture. The removed nail plate was shortened from the edges and repositioned over the area. The proximal nail fold stay sutures were removed and it was allowed to fall back in place. It was sutured on both sides with the lateral nail fold with non-absorbable sutures, avoiding suturing of the nail plate (Fig. 12.5). Tourniquet was removed, pressure hemostasis was secured and antiseptic dressing was done. The patient was advised post-operative analgesics for a week along with daily dressing change. The nail fold sutures were removed at 1 week.

Fig. 12.3a Proximal partial
nail plate avulsion and
retraction of the nail fold
exposes a large lesion
involving the nail bed

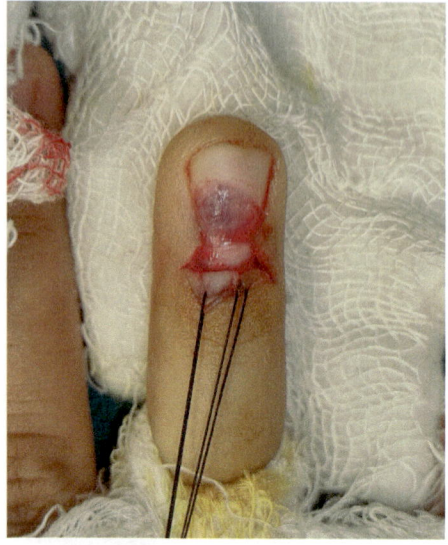

Fig. 12.3b Upon dissection,
a large jelly like mass,
suggestive of a glomus tumor,
is removed

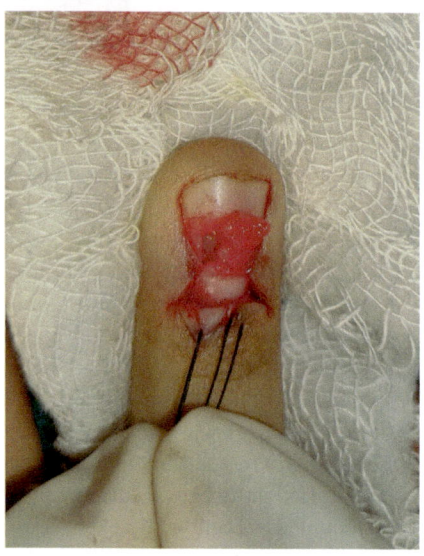

Histopathology of the excised specimen showed a well-circumscribed tumour composed of branching vascular channels, surrounded and separated by nests of monomorphic round cells with regular nuclei and eosinophilic cytoplasm, suggestive of a glomus tumor. The intervening stroma showed myxoid changes. Postoperative recovery was uneventful with regrowth of normal nail plate by 6 months. There was no residual pain, discoloration, or onycholysis.

Fig. 12.3c Excised tumor
specimen

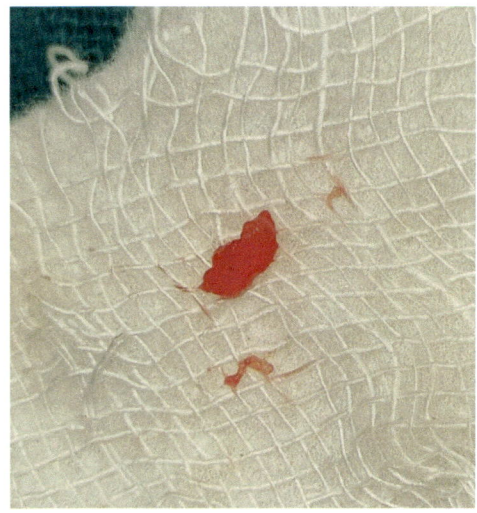

Fig. 12.3d Large nail bed
defect after tumor resection

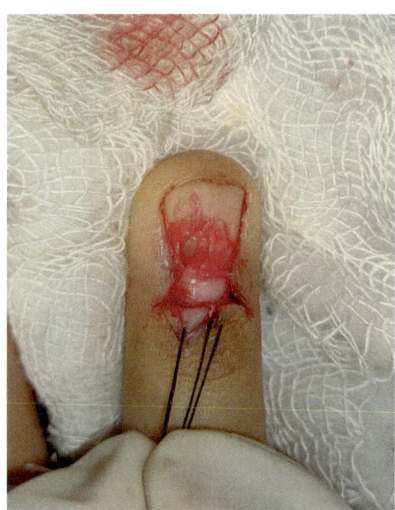

Discussion

A localised bluish discoloration of a nail is most commonly associated with a subungual hematoma as one of the acute causes [1, 5]. However, in cases with longstanding localised bluish discoloration, other causes, especially subungual tumors,
should always be assessed for. A painful bluish discoloration can point both towards
a subungual hematoma and a glomus tumor, but the intense pulsating pain and pin-
point tenderness in our case, made us suspect the diagnosis of glomus tumor [6, 7].

There are multiple causes of painful nails. An acronym ("GIFTED KID") suggested by Fonia and Richert is useful in this context [6]. The causes include G

Fig. 12.4 Intra-operative onychoscopy showing normal pink nail bed and paler nail matrix. No areas of bluish discoloration or prominent vasculature identified

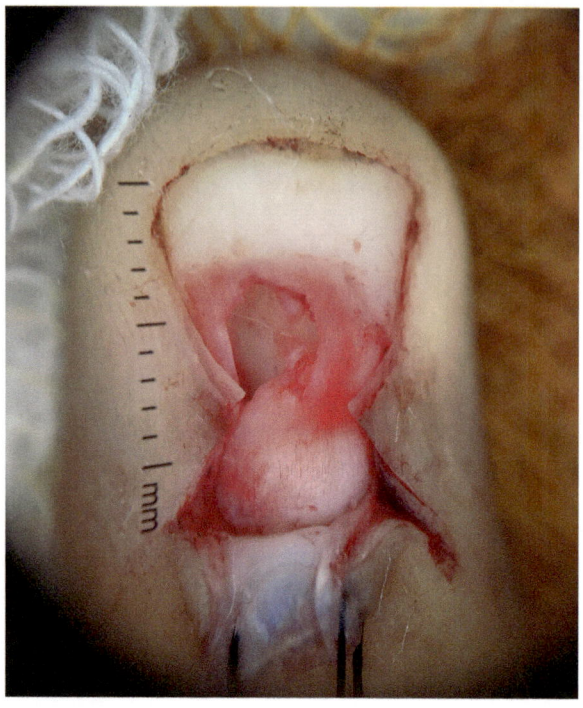

(Glomus tumor), I (Infections including acute paronychia, herpetic whitlow or non-dermatophyte onychomycosis), F (Foreign body insertion), T (traumatic causes including a subungual hematoma or subungual inclusion cysts), E (enchondroma), D (various Drugs including retinoids, chemotherapeutic agents like taxanes), K (subungual Keratoacanthoma), I (cold exposure leading to frostbite, expressed as Ice), D (gout, expressed as Dropping of urate crystals in the periungual and joint area). Among these, the intense pulsating pain, along with pin-point tenderness (also known as Love's pin test) is always in favour of a glomus tumor [7].

Bluish discoloration of the nail bed due to a subungual hematoma tends to change morphology with time. It is often a result of trauma (noticed or unnoticed) [1]. Common causes include direct trauma, like dropping something on the digit, falling or tripping, or catching the finger in a door. In these cases, the hematoma is fast to appear and can be quite symptomatic. Bleeding into the nail folds may also be seen, where it is easier to recognise due to the typical peripheral fading and color changes of a bruise. Repeated minor trauma like ill-fitting shoes, hiking downhill, active sports involving kicking, sharp turns or rapid movements etc. can also produce a subungual hematoma. The correlation with trauma may be difficult to make in such cases, and it is often noticed incidentally as it tends to be asymptomatic.

Glomus tumours are hamartomas of the glomus bodies [7]. These are the normal neuromyoarterial apparatus, seen much more commonly in the acral areas, especially digits, as they enable temperature control. Around 75% of glomus tumors

Fig. 12.5 Closure of the surgical wound with repositioning of the avulsed nail plate

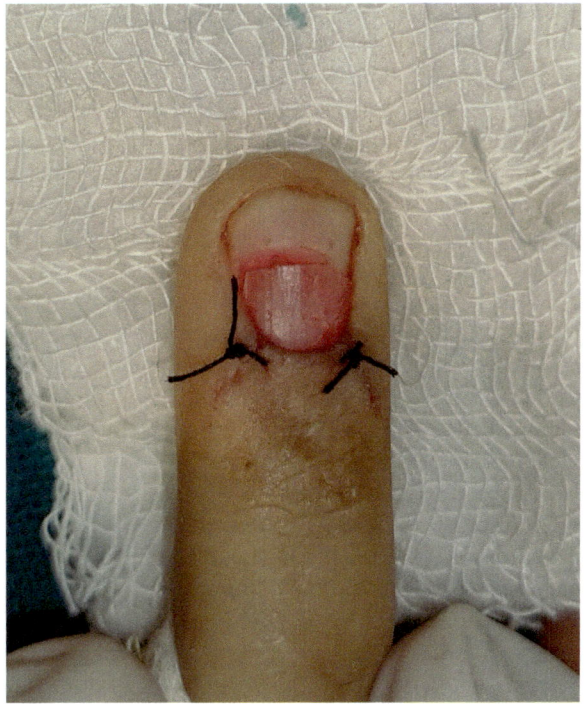

occur in the hand as these have a large number of glomus bodies [7]. Of these, roughly 65% are reported in the fingertips, especially subungually. Diagnostic delays are common as patients present with pain and there are no specific nail changes. Subungual glomus tumours characteristically present with paroxysmal pain, cold sensitivity and pin point tenderness [8]. A female preponderance has been reported [8]. Subungual glomus tumors are often difficult to visualise clinically. Nail discoloration (68.8% cases) and nail plate deformity (37.5% lesions) may be seen [8]. They are rarely palpable due to their size and location. Hence, imaging studies may be considered necessary to ensure precise localisation as it enables presurgical planning for precise excision and least collateral damage [9].

The clinical presentation may often reflect the location of the tumor. Isolated longitudinal erythronychia, with or without a distal splitting of the nail plate indicates a nail matrix tumor [10]. Longitudinal leukonychia has also been described, depending on the type of matrix lesion. Interestingly, some lesions may present with alternate red and white bands with distal 'V'-shaped notch. This has been termed as "candy-cane nails" and was classically associated with Darier disease [11]. It has been attributed to dilatation and compression of local vascular pattern caused by the mamillated surface of the tumour, as was seen in our case, where the tumor came out as a jelly like mass. This results in alternating erythronychia and apparent leukonychia, as matricial involvement gives rise to both splitting and subtle thinning of the nail plate causing erythematous streaks [10]. In the case of nail bed location, the mamillated tumor surface can give rise to localised areas of different color. In general, the more distally the tumour is located, the fewer defects are seen in the nail plate. Such a location, especially in the nail bed, is associated with diffuse erythronychia. Our patient had a bluish discoloration, which is not commonly described.

Onychoscopy was useful in confirming the diagnosis in our case. Onychoscopic features of subungual hematoma include purple-black colour (53%) as the most common colour change and homogenous pattern as the most common pattern [12]. A blue-white colour may also be seen in upto 26% lesions. Nail plate shows the presence of granular leukonychia in 19% lesions [12]. Upto 53% lesions may show a globular pattern, while 30% lesions show a 'streaks' pattern, which is the most distinctive feature for subungual hematoma. Peripheral fading of color, with typical color changes of a hematoma maybe present in upto 30% of the lesions. A periungual haemorrhage may also be seen occasionally. Onychoscopic features of glomus tumor are also distinctive [10]. Infact, they offer a valid clue towards the location of the tumor in the nail matrix or the nail bed [10]. Ill-defined, erythematous structureless areas interspersed with bluish-purple or reddish areas is typical of a subungual glomus tumor, especially of the nail bed. Changes in the nail plate in the form of distal onycholysis, longitudinal erythronychia or leukonychia, onychorrhexis, etc. are often a result of nail matrix tumors. Longitudinal bands of erythronychia interspersed with whitish areas (candy-cane appearance) is a change seen with nail matrix glomus tumors. Broader bands often suggest a larger lesion. Poorly focussed vessels (ramified telangiectatic vessels), distortion of the regular shape of lunula, or capillary rarefaction in proximal nail fold are seen with larger matrix lesions. Intraoperative onychooscopy can also show the same ramified blood vessels and bluish vascular blush which are helpful in defining the surgical margins as well as assessing for any residual lesion.

Being a painful nail tumor, the glomus significantly compromises the quality of life of its sufferer. The treatment is surgical excision, and dermatosurgeons need to be conversant with the surgical techniques used. A proper technique is important for preventing postoperative nail deformity, scarring, or tumor recurrence [7]. As discussed above, the location can be deduced on the basis of clinical examination, onychoscopy, and imaging. Depending on it, the best surgical approach should be planned which provides good visualization and prevent snail deformity at the same time. Clinically, Love's pin test can help localize the involved area and most of the patients are able to do this if counseled properly. Radiological investigation of choice is MRI which can pick up even very small lesions, as well as sister lesions which may not be very symptomatic [13].

Various surgical approaches have been highlighted for glomus excision, however, the transungual approach (requiring removal of overlying nail plate) is the most commonly used and effective method [7]. This was the method used in this case. The avulsion of the nail plate should be kept partial (lateral partial or proximal partial- depending on requirement). The lateral subungual approach, aimed at preserving the nail unit, is technically more difficult. It is also difficult to reach the more centrally located glomus tumors through this approach.

To prevent tumor recurrence, it is important to clearly visualize the complete lesion while dissecting it. This may take a few minutes to completely outline the extent. One may even need to avulse more nail than originally planned. However, in-toto resection minimises chances of recurrence. Sharp dissection at any stage may transect the tumor, leaving behind remnants which can be later responsible for recurrence of pain. After tumor excision and approximation of the surgical defect, a repositioning the removed nail plate in-situ should be attempted. It provides the best biological dressing for the exposed nail bed. The nail plate should be trimmed from edges (to prevent subungual seroma formation) and replaced over the exposed nail bed. It may be secured in position, if required, with 2–0 non-absorbable suture, removed after a week. Generally, the repositioned nail plate falls off; however, it still aids a faster regeneration of the nail bed epithelium, prevents formation of adhesions, and development of split nail or pterygium.

To conclude, a bluish painful discoloration of the nail should suggest a subungual glomus tumor. The post-operative outcomes depend entirely on the pre-operative workup and per-operative technique. Hence, none of these should be taken lightly. With proper planning and resources, the chances of scarring, disfigurement, incomplete resection, or reappearance of symptoms in a subungual glomus tumor, can be largely prevented.

Key Points

1. Subungual glomus tumour may occasionally present with a localised blue discoloration.
2. Presence of localised pain is strongly suggestive of a glomus, helping rule out other differential diagnoses.
3. Surgical excision should be carefully planned depending the localisation of the tumour.
4. With proper technique of transungual excision and post-operative nail plate repositioning, the chances of scarring, disfigurement, incomplete resection, or recurrence can be minimised.

References

1. Akella A, Daniel AR, Gould MB, Mangal R, Ganti L. Subungual Hematoma. Cureus. 2023;15(11):e48952.
2. Fox JD, Baker JA, Tosti A. Chromonychia in an asymptomatic vitamin consumer. Skin Appendage Disord. 2016;1(3):131–3.
3. Whelton MJ, Pope FM. Azure lunules in argyria. Corneal changes resembling Kayser-Fleischer rings. Arch Intern Med. 1968;121:267–9.
4. Weinberg LS, Arreola A, Mervak JE. Gray-blue discoloration of the proximal nail beds. JAAD Case Rep. 2023;35:126–8.

5. Singal A, Bisherwal K. Melanonychia: etiology, diagnosis, and treatment. Indian Dermatol Online J. 2020;11(1):1–11.
6. Fonia A, Richert B. Onychalgia causes and mechanisms: the "GIFTED KID" and the "FOMITE". Skin Appendage Disord. 2020;6(2):77–87.
7. Grover C, Khurana A, Jain R, Rathi V. Transungual surgical excision of subungual glomus tumour. J Cutan Aesthet Surg. 2013;6(4):196–203.
8. Singal A, Bisherwal K, Agrawal S, Bhat S, Diwakar P. Clinico-epidemiological profile and management outcome of subungual digital glomus tumor-Indian experience. Dermatol Ther. 2022;35(10):e15745.
9. Baek HJ, Lee SJ, Cho KH, et al. Subungual tumors: clinicopathologic correlation with US and MR imaging findings. Radiographics. 2010;30:1621–36.
10. Grover C, Jayasree P, Kaliyadan F. Clinical and onychoscopic characteristics of subungual glomus tumor: a cross-sectional study. Int J Dermatol. 2021 Jun;60(6):693–702.
11. Halteh P, Jorizzo JL, Lipner SR. Darier disease: candy-cane nails and hyperkeratotic papules. Postgrad Med J. 2016;92:425–6.
12. Metin MS, Elmas ÖF. Dermoscopic diagnosis of subungual hematoma: new observations. Postepy Dermatol Alergol. 2020;37(4):490–4.
13. Grover C, Bansal S, Varma A, Jakhar D. Radiological imaging of nail disorders (PART II) – radiological features of nail disease. Indian Dermatol Online J. 2022;13(6):701–9.

Chapter 13
Darier Disease with V-Nicking of the Nails

Madelyn M. Class ⓘ**, David Smith, Ryan P. Johnson, Nadia Abidi,
Mary M. Braden, Farhaan Hafeez, and Andrew C. Krakowski** ⓘ

Abstract A 55-year-old male presented with a longstanding history of pruritic rash on his back and incidentally discovered V-nicking of his nails. Histologic examination of the rash was consistent with a diagnosis of Darier disease. Darier disease is a rare genetic disorder that occurs due to mutations in the *ATP2A2* gene. The disease typically presents in childhood with pruritic hyperkeratotic papules coalescing into plaques in a seborrheic distribution. Nail abnormalities (such as V-nicking, brittle nails, and candy cane nails) are common.

Keywords Darier disease · V-nicking of nails · ATP2A2 gene mutation · Pruritic rash · Seborrheic distribution

Abbreviations/Acronyms

DD   Darier disease

M. M. Class (✉)
St. Luke's Department of Dermatology, St. Luke's University Health Network, Easton, PA, USA

Lewis Katz School of Medicine at Temple University, Bethlehem, PA, USA
e-mail: madelyn.class@temple.edu

D. Smith · R. P. Johnson · N. Abidi · M. M. Braden · F. Hafeez · A. C. Krakowski
St. Luke's Department of Dermatology, St. Luke's University Health Network, Easton, PA, USA
e-mail: david.smith@sluhn.org; ryan.johnson@sluhn.org; nadia.abidi@sluhn.org; mary.braden@sluhn.org; farhaan.hafeez@sluhn.org; andrew.krakowski@sluhn.org

© The Author(s), under exclusive license to Springer Nature Switzerland AG 2025
A. Tosti et al. (eds.), *Clinical Cases in Nail Disorders*, Clinical Cases in Dermatology, https://doi.org/10.1007/978-3-031-88642-3_13

Clinical Case

A 55-year-old male with a past medical history of hypertension and major depressive disorder presented to dermatology for a longstanding history of pruritic rash affecting his back in a "seborrheic distribution" (Fig. 13.1). He reported the rash had occurred since early adolescence and recurred more frequently—and was more bothersome—over the summer months. On physical exam, pinkish-tan crusted papules coalescing into near-confluent plaques were noted on the upper- and mid-back. "V-nicking" of the patient's nails was discovered on exam (Fig. 13.2). Upon further questioning, the patient revealed a history of "fragile nails" and a family history of similar skin and nail symptoms in his mother. Darier disease (DD) was suspected, and histologic examination of a central back punch biopsy demonstrated suprabasal clefts with acantholytic dyskeratosis, confirming the diagnosis.

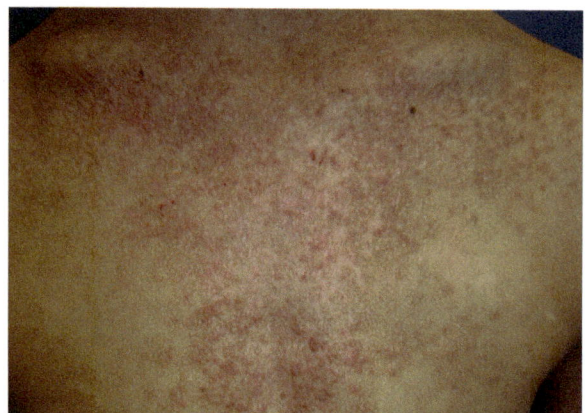

Fig. 13.1 Patient's upper- and mid-back with pinkish-tan papules coalescing into near-confluent plaques. (Source: Andrew C. Krakowski, MD)

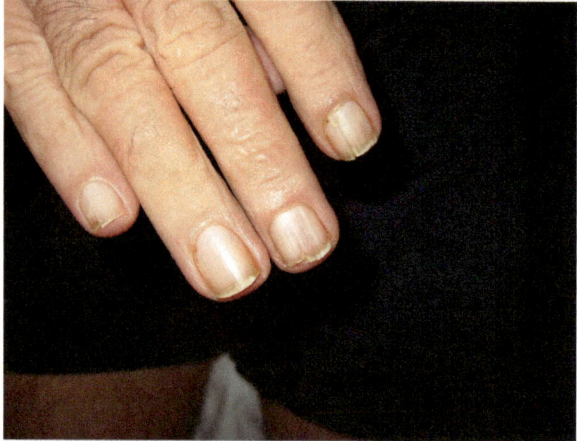

Fig. 13.2 Patient's right dorsal hand revealing V-nicking of the distal second, third, and fifth fingernails. (Source: Andrew C. Krakowski, MD)

What Is Your Diagnosis?

Diagnosis: Darier disease with V-nicking of the nails.

Differential diagnosis: Grover's disease, seborrheic dermatitis, Hailey-Hailey disease, confluent reticulate papillomatosis, pemphigus foliaceous, acne vulgaris, prurigo pigmentosa, reticulate erythematous mucinous syndrome, epidermodysplasia verruciformis, brittle nail syndrome, lichen planus.

Diagnosis

Darier disease with V-nicking of the nails.

Discussion

Darier disease (also known as "keratosis follicularis," "dyskeratosis follicularis," and "Darier-White disease") is a rare genetic disorder that occurs secondary to mutations in the *ATP2A2* gene [1, 2]. The *ATP2A2* gene encodes the sarco/endoplasmic reticulum Ca2+ adenosine triphosphatase isoform 2 (SERCA2), a P-type calcium ATPase [2]. SERCA2 maintains low calcium concentrations in the cytosol of keratinocytes, which is necessary for proper desmoplakin, a protein involved in desmosomal adhesions, function [1]. When mutated, abnormal SERCA2 function leads to epidermal dyskeratosis and acantholysis [1, 2].

Clinically, DD presents with hyperkeratotic papules coalescing into plaques in a "seborrheic" distribution that may affect the face, chest, back, and scalp [2]. Onset is typically in late-childhood/adolescence. Lesions are often pruritic and frequently become secondarily infected, leading to a strong malodor [2]. High temperatures, ultra-violet radiation, and mechanical irritation are known to exacerbate cutaneous DD symptoms [2, 3]. Nail abnormalities are common and may include brittle nails, V-nicking, and alternating longitudinal red and white bands more commonly referred to as "candy cane" nails [1, 2, 4]. In addition to the cutaneous findings of DD, neuropsychiatric disorders such as mood disorders and epilepsy are more highly associated with the condition [5, 6]. The *ATP2A2* gene is also expressed in the brain, suggesting that abnormal calcium homeostasis in the brain may play a direct role in terms of DD patients manifesting neuropsychiatric comorbidities [5, 6].

There is currently no cure or consensus treatment for DD; however, several different treatment approaches have been recommended for symptom management, including avoidance of exacerbating factors, oral retinoids, topical retinoids, 5-fluorouracil, surgical excision, dermabrasion, laser abrasion, among others [3].

Key Points

1. The combination of a papular, pruritic rash of seborrheic areas, along with V-nicking of the distal fingernails, should raise suspicion for Darier disease.
2. Darier disease is a rare genetic disorder of autosomal dominant inheritance that affects the *ATP2A2* gene, which encodes the sarco/endoplasmic reticulum Ca2+ adenosine triphosphatase isoform 2 (SERCA2), resulting in skin, nail, and neuropsychiatric abnormalities.

References

1. Bae-Harboe YSC, Mirzabeigi M, Gilchrest BA. Nail dystrophy and multiple hyperkeratotic papules on the face and neck. JAAD. 2013;69(5):847–9. https://doi.org/10.1016/j.jaad.2012.07.031.
2. Takagi A, Kamijo M, Ikeda S. Darier disease. J Dermatol. 2016;43(3):275–9. https://doi.org/10.1111/1346-8138.13230.
3. Haber RN, Dib NG. Management of Darier disease: a review of the literature and update. Indian J Dermatol Venereol Leprol. 2021;87(1):14–21. https://doi.org/10.25259/IJDVL_963_19.
4. Lipner SR, Scher RK. Evaluation of nail lines: color and shape hold clues. Cleve Clin J Med. 2016;83(5):385–91. https://doi.org/10.3949/ccjm.83a.14187.
5. Gordon-Smith K, Jones LA, Burge SM, et al. The neuropsychiatric phenotype in Darier disease. Br J Dermatol. 2010;163(3):515–22. https://doi.org/10.1111/j.1365-2133.2010.09834.x.
6. Jacobsen NJ, Lyons I, Hoogendoorn B, et al. ATP2A2 mutations in Darier's disease and their relationship to neuropsychiatric phenotypes. Hum Mol Genet. 1999;8(9):1631–6. https://doi.org/10.1093/hmg/8.9.1631.

Chapter 14
Koenen's Tumors (Periungual Angiofibromas)

David Smith, Madelyn M. Class ⓘ**, Ryan P. Johnson, Nadia Abidi,**
Laura Huang, and Andrew C. Krakowski ⓘ

Abstract A 60-year-old female presented with angiofibromas on her face and oral mucosa along with periungual angiofibromas (Koenen's tumors) on her fingers bilaterally. She did not have hypomelanotic macules, fibrous cephalic plaques, or Shagreen patches. Imaging revealed an enhancing brain tuber and multiple cysts in her kidneys bilaterally. The patient met criteria for a diagnosis of tuberous sclerosis complex. Tuberous sclerosis complex is a genetic disorder that involves the growth of hamartomas in any organ system due to inactivating mutations in the TSC1 and/ or TSC2 genes. The presence of periungual/ungual angiofibromas should prompt an evaluation for tuberous sclerosis complex.

Keywords Tuberous sclerosis · Periungual angiofibromas · Koenen's tumors · Hamartomas · Ungual angiofibromas

Abbreviations/Acronyms

TSC   tuberous sclerosis complex
mTOR   mammalian target of rapamycin

D. Smith (✉) · R. P. Johnson · N. Abidi · L. Huang · A. C. Krakowski
St. Luke's Department of Dermatology; St. Luke's University Health Network, Easton, PA, USA
e-mail: david.smith@sluhn.org; ryan.johnson@sluhn.org; nadia.abidi@sluhn.org; laura.huang@sluhn.org; andrew.krakowski@sluhn.org

M. M. Class
St. Luke's Department of Dermatology; St. Luke's University Health Network, Easton, PA, USA

Lewis Katz School of Medicine at Temple University, Bethlehem, PA, USA
e-mail: madelyn.class@temple.edu

© The Author(s), under exclusive license to Springer Nature Switzerland AG 2025
A. Tosti et al. (eds.), *Clinical Cases in Nail Disorders*, Clinical Cases in Dermatology, https://doi.org/10.1007/978-3-031-88642-3_14

Clinical Case

A 60-year-old woman with a past medical history of nonalcoholic steatohepatitis, anxiety, depression, stage 3 chronic kidney disease, and hypertension presented to dermatology for a seborrheic keratosis on her abdomen. During her full body skin exam, papules were noted on her face, fingers (Fig. 14.1), and oral mucosa that resembled angiofibromas and were later confirmed as such via skin and oral mucosal biopsies. Hypomelanotic macules, fibrous cephalic plaques, and Shagreen patches were not noted—even under Wood's lamp exam. Brain imaging demonstrated a 1-cm focus of enhancement within the left frontal lobe for which an enhancing tuber, infection, or inflammatory etiology could not be excluded. Chest and abdominal imaging studies revealed multiple cysts in the upper poles of her bilateral kidneys, along with interstitial lung disease. Echocardiogram showed no evidence of cardiac rhabdomyomas. The patient denied any history of seizures.

What Is Your Diagnosis?

Diagnosis: Koenen's tumors (periungual angiofibromas) in the setting of tuberous sclerosis complex (TSC)

Differential diagnosis: Multiple Endocrine Neoplasia Type 1, verruca vulgaris, subungual exostosis, myxoid cyst, acquired digital fibrokeratoma, Cowden disease, Birt-Hogg-Dubé Syndrome

Fig. 14.1 Patient's right hand revealing Koenen's tumors (periungual angiofibromas) on the fourth and fifth digits. (Source: Madelyn M. Class)

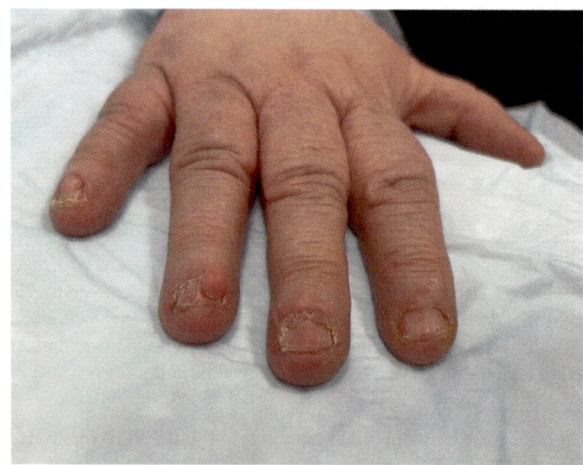

Diagnosis

Koenen's tumors (periungual angiofibromas) in the setting of TSC

Discussion

TSC is a rare genetic disease that involves the growth of benign tumors—hamarto-mas—of any organ system [1]. The disorder arises secondary to inactivating gene mutations in the TSC1 and/or TSC2 genes, leading to dysregulated mammalian target of rapamycin (mTOR) signaling and unregulated cellular proliferation [2, 3]. Presentation varies greatly among affected individuals, with unpredictable organ system involvement, size and number of hamartomas, and effect on quality of life [1]. The greatest morbidity and mortality associated with the condition involves the neurologic and neuropsychiatric manifestations because brain involvement can cause symptoms such as seizures, developmental delay, anxiety, mood disorders, obstructive hydrocephalus, and even death [2].

TSC can be diagnosed clinically or through genetic testing. Clinical diagnosis requires two major features of TSC or one major feature with two minor features [4]. The major criteria include: hypomelanotic macules ($\geq$ 3; at least 5 mm diame-ter); angiofibromas ($\geq$3) or fibrous cephalic plaque; ungual fibromas ($\geq$2); Shagreen patch; multiple retinal hamartomas; multiple cortical tubers and/or radial migration lines; subependymal nodule ($\geq$2); subependymal giant cell astrocytoma; cardiac rhabdomyoma; lymphangiomyomatosis; and angiomyolipomas ($\geq$2) [4]. The minor criteria include: "Confetti" skin lesions; dental enamel pits ($\geq$3); intraoral fibromas ($\geq$2); retinal achromic patch; multiple renal cysts; nonrenal hamartomas; and scle-rotic bone lesions [4]. A pathogenic variant in TSC1 or TSC2 identified through genetic testing is also sufficient for a TSC diagnosis, even without clinical findings [4]. Interestingly, seizure history, which is common in many patients with TSC, is not part of the diagnostic criteria. Our patient met diagnostic criteria with $\geq$3 angio-fibromas (major criterion), $\geq$2 ungual fibromas (major criterion), $\geq$2 intraoral fibro-mas (minor criterion), and multiple renal cysts (minor criterion). Prior to the currently accepted diagnostic criteria, findings such as a single ungual fibroma or multiple angiofibromas were considered pathognomonic for TSC [5]. As many of the diagnostic criteria are cutaneous and often the first clinical features to develop, dermatologists must remain vigilant to help make an early diagnosis of TSC [6]. Management should be "multidisciplinary" with early referrals to neurology, oph-thalmology, cardiology, pulmonology, nephrology, psychiatry, and dentistry. Patients and their families should also be offered genetic counseling.

Treatment is mostly symptomatic, with surgery for removal of problematic ham-artomas or with medications such as anti-epileptics or mood stabilizers [3]. More recently, studies looking at the effect of topical and systemic mTOR inhibitors on TSC manifestations have been underway and show promise for the future treatment of TSC [2, 3]. Currently 2% sirolimus gel has been approved by the U.S. Food and Drug Administration for topical treatment of facial angiofibromas, in patients 6 years of age and older. Our patient deferred further treatment at this time.

Key Points

1. A patient can meet criteria for TSC diagnosis through cutaneous findings alone.
2. Nail examination revealing ungual angiofibromas should prompt a comprehensive evaluation for tuberous sclerosis.

References

1. Curatolo P, Bombardieri R, Jozwiak S. Tuberous sclerosis. Lancet. 2008;372(9639):657–68. https://doi.org/10.1016/S0140-6736(08)61279-9.
2. Salussolia CL, Klonowska K, Kwiatkoski DJ, Sahin M. Genetic etiologies, diagnosis, and treatment of tuberous sclerosis complex. Annu Rev Genomics Hum Genet. 2019;20:217–40. https://doi.org/10.1146/annurev-genom-083118-015354.
3. Kohrman MH. Emerging treatments in the management of tuberous sclerosis complex. Pediatr Neurol. 2012;46(5):267–75. https://doi.org/10.1016/j.pediatrneurol.2012.02.015.
4. Northrup H, Aronow ME, Bebin EM, et al. Updated international tuberous sclerosis complex diagnostic criteria and surveillance and management recommendations. Pediatr Neurol. 2021;123:50–66. https://doi.org/10.1016/j.pediatrneurol.2021.07.011.
5. Schwartz RA, Fernández G, Kotulska K, Jóźwiak S. Tuberous sclerosis complex: advances in diagnosis, genetics, and management. J Am Acad Dermatol. 2007;57(2):189–202. https://doi.org/10.1016/j.jaad.2007.05.004.
6. Tsao H, Luo S. Chapter 61: Neurofibromatosis and tuberous sclerosis complex. In: Bolognia JL, Schaffer JV, Cerroni L, et al., editors. Dermatology. 4th ed. Elsevier; 2017. p. 985–1003.

Chapter 15
Lichen Striatus Affecting the Nail

Madelyn M. Class (iD)**, Taylor Jones, Stephen Senft, Alan Westheim, Laura Huang, Nadia Abidi, Ryan P. Johnson, and Andrew C. Krakowski** (iD)

Abstract Two patients presented with linear pink papules on a dorsal digit along with associated nail findings. An 8-year-old male had longitudinal splitting of the left third nail, while a 7-year-old male had longitudinal ridging of the left first nail. Both were diagnosed with lichen striatus with nail involvement. Lichen striatus is a benign dermatologic condition of unknown etiology that mainly affects children. It typically presents with an asymptomatic papular rash in a linear distribution. If the cutaneous eruption is on a digit, there can be associated nail changes. Nail findings include longitudinal ridging or splitting. The cutaneous findings typically self-resolve within 2 years, while the nail findings may take up to 5 years to self-resolve.

Keywords Lichen striatus · Linear pink papules · Longitudinal splitting · Longitudinal ridging · Linear rash

M. M. Class (✉)
St. Luke's Department of Dermatology, St. Luke's University Health Network, Easton, PA, USA

Lewis Katz School of Medicine at Temple University, Bethlehem, PA, USA
e-mail: madelyn.class@temple.edu

T. Jones
West Virginia School of Osteopathic Medicine, Lewisburg, WV, USA
e-mail: tjones@osteo.wvsom.edu

S. Senft · A. Westheim · L. Huang · N. Abidi · R. P. Johnson · A. C. Krakowski
St. Luke's Department of Dermatology, St. Luke's University Health Network, Easton, PA, USA
e-mail: stephen.senft@sluhn.org; alan.westheim@sluhn.org; laura.huang@sluhn.org; nadia.abidi@sluhn.org; ryan.johnson@sluhn.org; andrew.krakowski@sluhn.org

© The Author(s), under exclusive license to Springer Nature Switzerland AG 2025
A. Tosti et al. (eds.), *Clinical Cases in Nail Disorders*, Clinical Cases in Dermatology, https://doi.org/10.1007/978-3-031-88642-3_15

Clinical Cases

1. An 8-year-old male with a past medical history of seasonal allergies and asthma presented to pediatric dermatology clinic for a 1-month history of a pruritic rash of his left third digit. On exam, linear pink papules with excoriations on the left dorsal lateral third digit were noted, along with longitudinal splitting of the associated central lateral nail (Figs. 15.1a and 15.1b). The diagnosis of lichen striatus of the digit and nail was made, and the patient was prescribed topical corticosteroids to help relieve the itch.

2. A 7-year-old male with a past medical history of anxiety presented to pediatric dermatology clinic for a 2-month history of an asymptomatic rash of his left dorsal first digit. On exam, pink papules in a linear distribution were noted along the length of his left dorsal first digit along with longitudinal ridging of the left lateral first fingernail (Figs. 15.2a and 15.2b). The diagnosis of lichen striatus of the digit was made. The patient and his family were reassured of the benign course of the diagnosis, and they were instructed to follow up if the findings did not resolve within several years.

Fig. 15.1a Patient's left third digit with linearly-arranged pink eczematous papules and longitudinal splitting of the central lateral nail. (Source: Andrew C. Krakowski, MD)

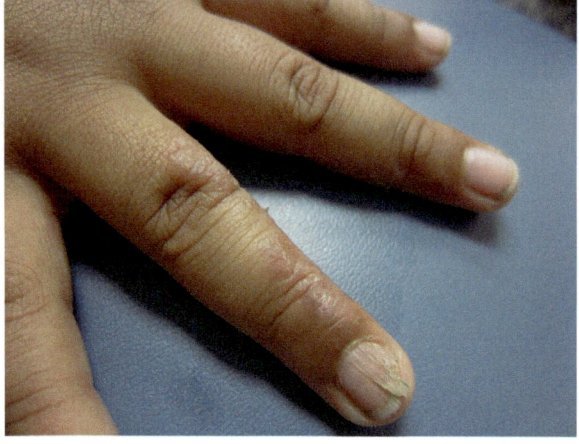

Fig. 15.1b Patient's dorsal left lateral third digit, revealing linearly-arranged pink eczematous papules along the length of the digit with longitudinal splitting of the nail. (Source: Andrew C. Krakowski, MD)

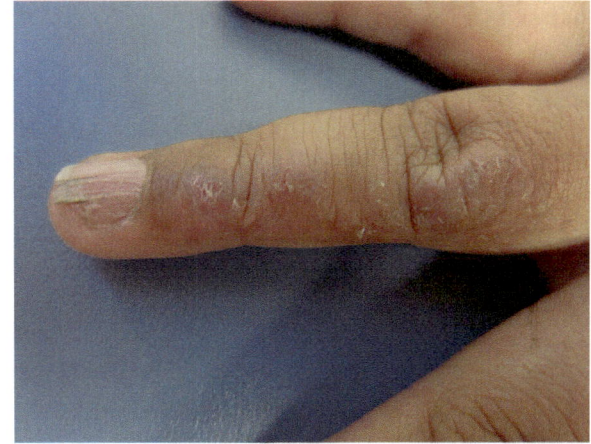

Fig. 15.2a Patient's left dorsal first digit with linearly-arranged, pink, lichenoid papules along the length of the digit with longitudinal ridging of the left lateral first fingernail. (Source: Andrew C. Krakowski, MD)

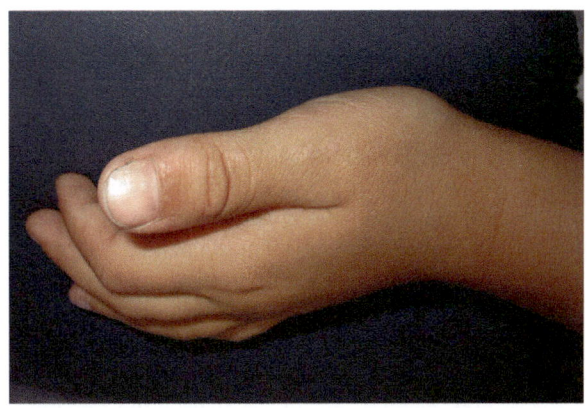

Fig. 15.2b Patient's left first fingernail revealing longitudinal ridging in alignment with linearly-arranged, pink, lichenoid papules of skin. (Source: Andrew C. Krakowski, MD)

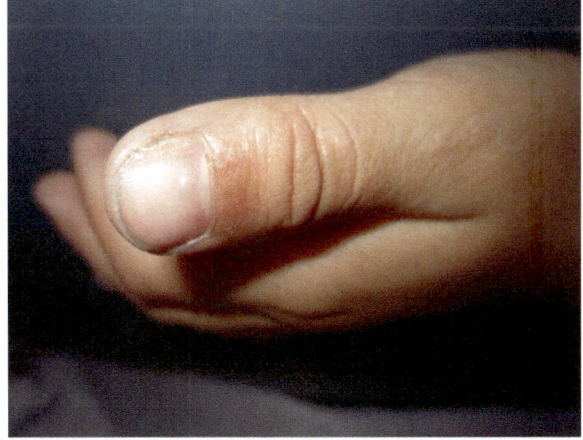

What Is Your Diagnosis?

Diagnosis: Lichen striatus with nail involvement.

Differential diagnosis: lichen planus, inflammatory linear verrucous epidermal nevus, linear psoriasis, median nail dystrophy of Heller, linear porokeratosis, linear lichen sclerosus, nevus unius lateris, linear Darier disease, lichen nitidus, lichen simplex chronicus, verruca vulgaris.

Diagnosis

Lichen striatus with nail involvement.

Discussion

Lichen striatus is an uncommon dermatologic condition that mainly affects children and typically erupts as raised pink-colored, lichenoid or eczematous papules [1]. These lesions transform over time to become linear and follow the distribution of Blaschko's lines [2]. The most common areas to be involved include the extremities, followed by the trunk, buttocks, face, and neck [3]. Less commonly, lichen striatus may affect the nails causing them to thicken, become rigid, and potentially even fall off [1]. Nail involvement may present with or without associated skin involvement and may be the only sign of lichen striatus [4]. This diagnosis should be suspected when a patient presents with lateral or medial involvement in only one nail [4, 5].

In the reported case presentations, lichen striatus of the nail was diagnosed on the basis of pink papules in a linear distribution affecting one digit and its associated nail. One patient was otherwise completely asymptomatic, while the other experienced only mild pruritus.

Lichen striatus has an unknown etiology, though environmental, cutaneous injury, viral infection, hypersensitivity, and genetic factors are thought to play a role [5]. Atopy, where patients have a predisposition to allergic conditions such as eczema and asthma, seems to positively correlate. There has also been proposed connections with pregnancy, vitiligo, and the drugs adalimumab and etanercept [1]. There have been cases reported in children living in shared environments, suggesting an environmental component [1]. Histology of lichen striatus shows a lichenoid infiltrate in the epidermis, which is typically acanthotic [1]. It is thought that inflammation of the nail matrix is T-cell mediated causing keratin production in the nail plate to be defective [5]. The defective keratin production is believed to be responsible for the abnormalities seen in the nail with lichen striatus [5].

Other dermatologic conditions need to be ruled out prior to making the diagnosis of lichen striatus. Common differential diagnoses include, but are not limited to, nevus unius lateris, inflammatory linear verrucous epidermal nevus, median nail dystrophy of Heller, linear lichen sclerosus, linear Darier disease, lichen nitidus, lichen planus, lichen simplex chronicus, verruca vulgaris, linear psoriasis, and linear porokeratosis [1]. In some cases it may be difficult to distinguish lichen striatus from lichen planus as both can present with cutaneous and nail findings. Typically, lichen planus is characterized by pruritic papules/plaques that in rare instances are linear [6]. Nail involvement associated with lichen planus is infrequent but when present is most commonly melanonychia and/or onychorrhexis of multiple fingernails, often with toenail involvement as well [7]. In contrast, lichen striatus is commonly characterized by a nonpruritic, linearly distributed rash, with nail involvement that most commonly includes longitudinal ridging or splitting limited to one digit in close proximity to the cutaneous eruption [6, 8]. Histology can also help distinguish between these two conditions [6].

Lichen striatus typically resolves spontaneously within 6 months to 2 years [2]. However, nail involvement may extend that time period to up to 5 years [1, 2]. Once the condition resolves, the skin and nail typically heal without deformity [1]. While there is no specific treatment for lichen striatus, topical and intralesional steroids and tacrolimus 0.1% ointment have been used to treat affected skin and nails [2, 4, 9]. Alternative treatment includes oral cyclosporine [2].

Key Points

1. If a child presents with an asymptomatic, linear, papular rash of a single digit with nail involvement, lichen striatus with nail involvement should be high on the differential.
2. Lichen striatus is a self-resolving condition with an unknown etiology.

References

1. Charifa A, Jamil RT, Ramphul K. Lichen striatus. In: StatPearls [Internet]. StatPearls Publishing; 2023.
2. Liu ZR, Zhou Y, Liu MX, Wang XQ, Wang DG. Lichen striatus with nail involvement: two case reports. Int J Dermatol Venereol. 2021;4(4):254–6. https://doi.org/10.1097/JD9.0000000000000063.
3. Leung AKC, Leong KF, Barankin B. Lichen striatus with nail involvement in a 6-year-old boy. Case Rep Pediatr. 2020;2020:1494760. https://doi.org/10.1155/2020/1494760.
4. Kim M, Jung HY, Eun YS, Cho BK, Park HJ. Nail lichen striatus: report of seven cases and review of the literature. Int J Dermatol. 2015;54(11):1255–60. https://doi.org/10.1111/ijd.12643.
5. Das S, Adhicari P. Lichen striatus in children: a clinical study of ten cases with review of literature. Indian J Paediatr Dermatol. 2017;18(2):89–93. https://doi.org/10.4103/2319-7250.202997.

6. Pulgar F, Rivera R, Rodríguez-Peralto JL, Vanaclocha F. Lichen planus and lichen striatus: opposite ends of the same spectrum? Actas Dermosifiliogr (English Edition). 2009;100(10):915–7. https://doi.org/10.1016/s1578-2190(09)70569-4.
7. Wechsuruk P, Bunyaratavej S, Kiratiwongwan R, et al. Clinical features and treatment outcomes of nail lichen planus: a retrospective study. JAAD Case Rep. 2021;17:43–8. https://doi.org/10.1016/j.dcr.2021.09.015.
8. Jakhar D, Kaur I. Onychoscopy of nail involvement in lichen striatus. Indian Dermatol Online J. 2018;9(5):360–1. https://doi.org/10.4103/idoj.IDOJ_299_17.
9. Cheon DUK, Ro YS, Kim JE. Treatment of nail lichen striatus with intralesional steroid injection: a case report and literature review. Dermatol Ther. 2018;31(6):e12713. https://doi.org/10.1111/dth.12713.

Chapter 16
Hemorrhagic Onycholysis Secondary to Docetaxel

Anuj Kunadia ⓘ, Amanda Weissman ⓘ, and Jarad Levin ⓘ

Abstract A 67-year-old Black female undergoing chemotherapy with docetaxel presented with hemorrhagic onycholysis affecting all 20 nails. Physical examination revealed subungual hematomas, onycholysis, onychauxis, and nail plate loss. Fungal cultures were negative. This case highlights the rare but challenging adverse effect of taxane-induced hemorrhagic onycholysis.

Keywords Onycholysis · Docetaxel · Chemotherapy · Taxane · Onychauxis

Clinical Case

A 67-year-old Black female with a history of stage IVB uterine serous cancer, undergoing chemotherapy with carboplatin and docetaxel, presented as a new patient for nail dystrophy. She reported that her nails, which were previously normal before chemotherapy, had recently begun to change color, lift and fall off. This change affected all 20 nails. She noted peripheral neuropathy from her chemotherapy but denied other symptoms. Her self-management attempts included using over-the-counter antifungal polish, a 10-day course of cephalexin, and soaking the nails, none of which helped her condition. A scraping of the toenails and surrounding hyperkeratotic skin was sent for fungal culture, which yielded negative growth of fungal elements.

A. Kunadia (✉) · A. Weissman
Dermatology Resident, University of Oklahoma Department of Dermatology,
Oklahoma City, OK, USA
e-mail: anuj-kunadia@ouhsc.edu; amanda-weissman@ouhsc.edu

J. Levin
Dermatology Faculty, University of Oklahoma Department of Dermatology,
Oklahoma City, OK, USA
e-mail: jarad-levin@ouhsc.edu

© The Author(s), under exclusive license to Springer Nature
Switzerland AG 2025
A. Tosti et al. (eds.), *Clinical Cases in Nail Disorders*, Clinical Cases in
Dermatology, https://doi.org/10.1007/978-3-031-88642-3_16

Fig. 16.1 Reddish-brown subungual hematomas, onycholysis, onychauxis, and missing nail plates in a 67-year-old female being treated with docetaxel

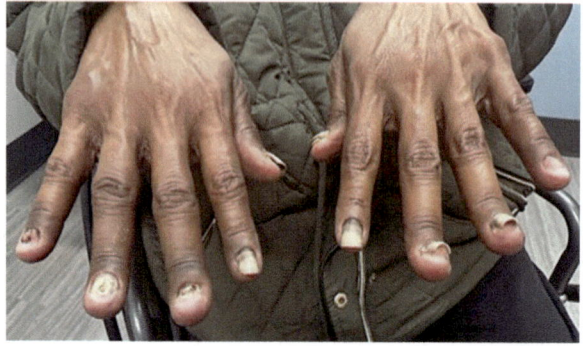

Physical exam findings included the absence of nail plates on the right lateral three nails and the left fifth finger, with hemorrhagic crusting over the nail bed. The remaining fingernails showed reddish-brown subungual hematomas, onycholysis, and some with onychauxis (Fig. 16.1). All ten toenails had reddish-brown subungual hematomas and onychauxis (Fig. 16.2).

Differential Diagnoses

The differential diagnosis for this patient included chemical exposure including nail cosmetics, inflammatory conditions such as psoriasis or lichen planus, infections such as dermatophytes causing onychomycosis, systemic diseases such as thyroid abnormalities, and medication induced onycholysis such as that associated with docetaxel or nonsteroidal anti-inflammatory drugs.

Diagnosis

Given the patient's clinical presentation and history, the final diagnosis was hemorrhagic onycholysis associated with docetaxel.

Discussion

This case illustrates hemorrhagic onycholysis associated with taxane chemotherapy, particularly docetaxel. Docetaxel and paclitaxel are the cytotoxic drugs most frequently associated with onycholysis [1]. Other agents previously

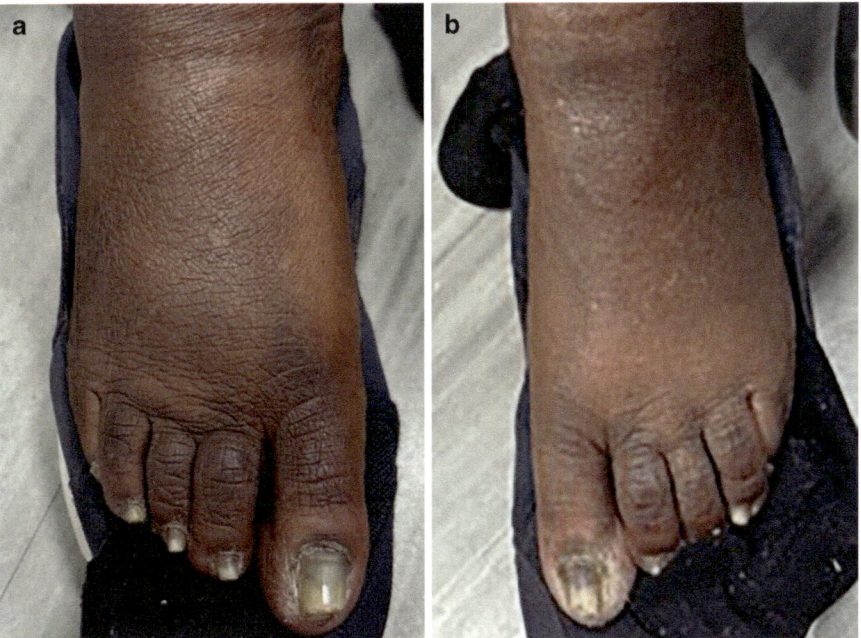

Fig. 16.2 (**a, b**) All of the patient's toenails exhibited reddish-brown discoloration and onychauxis

reported to cause onycholysis include doxorubicin, cyclophosphamide, etoposide, 5-fluorouracil, capecitabine, hydroxyurea, ixabepilone, and the combination of bleomycin plus vinblastine. Onycholysis may be a challenging adverse reaction for patients due to nail pain, jagged edges causing breakage, and cosmetic disfigurement. While there is no definitive treatment, the use of cryotherapy has shown limited evidence of benefiting affected patients. In one study, the use of a frozen glove on one hand of patients undergoing docetaxel chemotherapy significantly reduced nail side effects, with no onycholysis observed in the gloved hands compared to 22% in unprotected hands. Nail changes were absent in 89% of gloved hands versus 49% in unprotected hands [2]. Another study found limited efficacy of this method, with no significant differences in nail discoloration, loss, or ridging between gloved and non-gloved hands, and a high withdrawal rate of 60% due to patient discomfort, suggesting varied results and patient tolerance in different clinical settings [3]. As research continues, future studies may focus on optimizing the balance between efficacy and patient comfort in the use of cold therapies such as frozen gloves during chemotherapy, to find more applicable and patient-friendly solutions for managing this taxane-induced nail toxicity.

Key Points

- Chemotherapy, especially with the taxane class of chemotherapeutic agents like docetaxel, can lead to significant nail changes, including onycholysis, subungual hematomas, and onychauxis.
- Patients with hemorrhagic onycholysis associated with taxane chemotherapy may benefit from cryotherapy, such as using a frozen glove during chemotherapy. This has shown some promise in reducing nail side effects, but its effectiveness can vary, and patient comfort is a significant factor to consider when employing this treatment.

References

1. Wasner G, Hilpert F, Schattschneider J, Binder A, Pfisterer J, Baron R. Docetaxel-induced nail changes--a neurogenic mechanism: a case report. J Neurooncol. 2002;58(2):167–74. https://doi.org/10.1023/a:1016002329546.
2. Scotté F, Tourani JM, Banu E, et al. Multicenter study of a frozen glove to prevent docetaxel-induced onycholysis and cutaneous toxicity of the hand. J Clin Oncol. 2005;23(19):4424–9. https://doi.org/10.1200/JCO.2005.15.651.
3. Morrison A, Marshall-McKenna R, McFadyen AK, Hutchison C, Rice AM, Stirling L, McIlroy P, Macpherson IR. A randomised controlled trial of interventions for taxane-induced nail toxicity in women with early breast cancer. Sci Rep. 2022;12(1):11575. https://doi.org/10.1038/s41598-022-13327-6. PMID: 35798751; PMCID: PMC9262963

Chapter 17
A Case of Onychopapilloma Presenting as Longitudinal Erythronychia

Eden Axler ⓘ **and Shari R. Lipner** ⓘ

Abstract A 57-year-old male presented with a 5-year history of a red longitudinal band and splinter hemorrhages involving the left thumbnail. Physical examination showed longitudinal erythronychia and a distal subungual hyperkeratotic papule. Excision with histopathology showed focal hyperplasia, elongated rete ridges, onycholemmal keratinization, and vascular ectasia, consistent with an onychopapilloma. Longitudinal erythronychia has a broad differential, including benign and malignant conditions. In equivocal cases, diagnosis requires excision with histopathology.

Keywords Onychopapilloma · Longitudinal erythronychia · Nail tumor · Histopathology · Splinter hemorrhages

Clinical Case Description

A 57-year-old male, Fitzpatrick skin type II, presented with a 5-year history of a red band and "splinter" involving the left thumbnail. He reported that the band slowly widened over time and endorsed intermittent pain with pressure, but no cold-induced discomfort. He had a prior diagnosis of onychomycosis confirmed via nail clipping with histopathology showing hyphae and was treated with two separate courses of terbinafine treatment for 3 months each, with no change in the appearance of the nail. Physical examination of the left thumbnail showed a red longitudinal band with long splinter hemorrhages (Fig. 17.1). There was a hyperkeratotic papule subungally when viewed end on, that was enhanced with

E. Axler · S. R. Lipner (✉)
Department of Dermatology, Weill Cornell Medicine, New York, NY, USA
e-mail: Eda4007@med.cornell.edu; shl9032@med.cornell.edu

© The Author(s), under exclusive license to Springer Nature Switzerland AG 2025
A. Tosti et al. (eds.), *Clinical Cases in Nail Disorders*, Clinical Cases in Dermatology, https://doi.org/10.1007/978-3-031-88642-3_17

101

Fig. 17.1 Left thumbnail
with longitudinal
erythronychia and splinter
hemorrhages

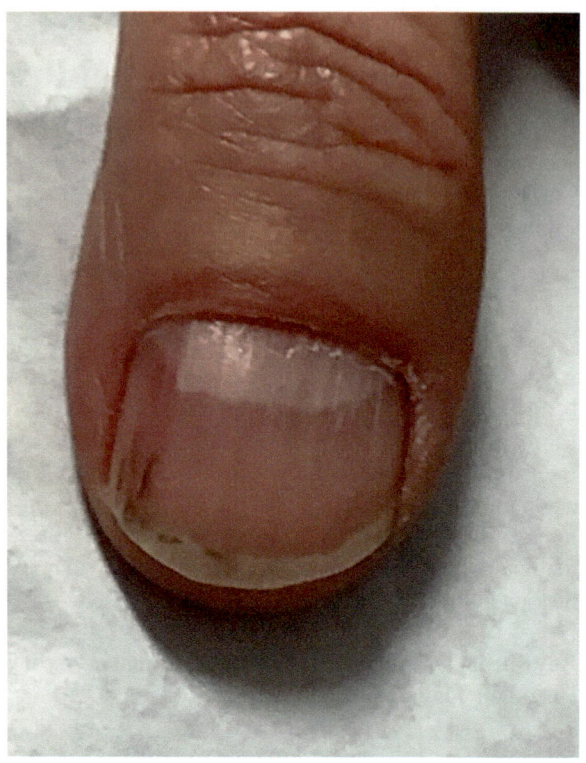

dermoscopy. Nail biopsy was recommended due to recent growth and associated pain.

An X-ray was performed, which was negative for bone erosion, which would have been supportive of a glomus tumor. A longitudinal excision was performed with histopathology showing a normal nail matrix that merged with the nail bed epithelium. The nail bed epithelium exhibited focal hyperplasia with elongated rete ridge-like or peg-like structures, indicative of acanthosis with focal dyskeratosis. Additionally, onycholemmal buds emanated from these structures, displaying a unique form of keratinization resembling onycholemmal keratinization, typically seen in the keratogenous zone of the nail matrix but observed in the nail bed in this case. The adjacent hyponychium appeared normal, while the subjacent corium exhibited signs of fibrosis. Notably, vascular ectasia was observed in areas of epithelial hyperplasia, potentially contributing to the redness observed (Fig. 17.2).

Fig. 17.2 (**a, b**)
Longitudinal excision of
nail bed, left thumbnail.
Nail bed epithelium
becomes hyperplastic with
elongated rete ridge-like or
peg-like structures as a
unique form of acanthosis
with focal dyskeratosis,
along with onycholemmal
buds emanating from these
elongated epithelial
structures. A (Left):
*Hematoxylin and eosin
stain 200X. B (Right):
Hematoxylin and eosin
stain 100X*

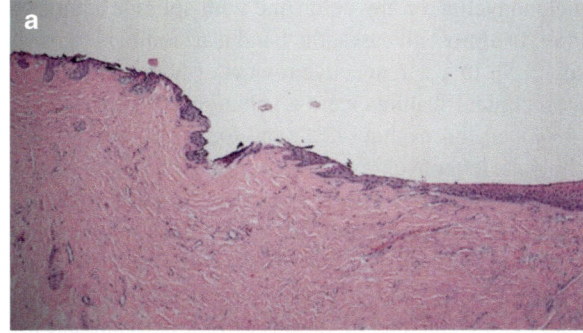

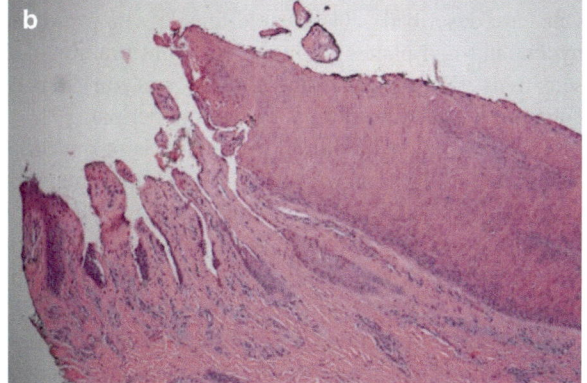

Differential Diagnosis

(a) Glomus tumor
(b) Scar
(c) Onychopapilloma
(d) Verruca Vulgaris
(e) Squamous Cell Carcinoma (SCC)

Correct Diagnosis

Onychopapilloma

Discussion

Onychopapilloma is a benign tumor of the nail bed and distal nail matrix [1]. The
most common presentation of onychopapilloma is longitudinal erythronychia.
Less common presentations include longitudinal leukonychia, longitudinal

melanonychia, or any color line with splinter hemorrhages, which may be short or long. In almost all cases, the band is accompanied by distal subungual hyperkeratosis [2, 3]. In a retrospective review of 50 onychopapilloma patients, the most common clinical features were a subungual hyperkeratotic mass (58%), distal fissures (46%), erythronychia (42%) and longitudinal ridging (42%). Less frequently, onycholysis, leukonychia, short splinter hemorrhages, melanonychia, and long splinter hemorrhages were observed [4]. Onychopapillomas are typically asymptomatic, but some patients may report that it interferes with daily activities, such as picking up small objects [5]. In a retrospective review of 68 patients with onychopapilloma, eight patients (15%) were asymptomatic, though functional problems including pain (41%), catching on fabrics (48%), or distal nail fragility (39%) were noted [6]. One case described a 74-year-old female who presented with longitudinal erythronychia and nail plate splitting of the right thumbnail. She reported throbbing and sensitivity. Biopsy with histopathology was consistent onychopapilloma with a concomitant traumatic neuroma, explaining her pain [7].

Onychoscopy is helpful in the diagnosis of onychopapilloma. In a retrospective review including 39 patients with onychopapilloma, the most common dermoscopic features were distal subungual hyperkeratosis (100%), splinter hemorrhage (69%), onycholysis (62%), a notch in the lunula (56%), macrolunula (31%), trailing lunula along the longitudinal band (21%), distal fissuring (15%), and punctiform hemorrhages (5%) [8].

A longitudinal band with a distal hyperkeratotic papule that is stable over time is most likely an onychopapilloma. No biopsy is necessary, and the patient may be followed longitudinally. A biopsy with histopathology is necessary for definitive diagnosis when there are atypical clinical features or evolution. Differential diagnosis of single digit longitudinal erythronychia includes glomus tumor, scar, verruca vulgaris, amelanotic melanoma, SCC, and malignant onychopapilloma. In a retrospective study of 15 onychopapilloma cases that underwent nail biopsy, histopathology of excisional specimens most commonly showed papillomatosis (87%), nail matrix metaplasia of nail bed (60%), subungual hyperkeratosis (53%) and hemorrhage (20%) [3]. Other features included parakeratosis, acanthosis, and keratinocyte multinucleation [3].

In a retrospective study of 61 monodactylous longitudinal erythronychia cases confirmed histologically, onychopapilloma was the diagnosis in 67% of cases, with SCC in situ in 4.9%, and amelanotic melanoma in 1.6% [9]. Malignant onychopapilloma is a rare variant of onychopapilloma, with 5 cases reported to date [10–12]. In a retrospective study of 91 histopathologically confirmed onychopapillomas, there were 3 malignant onychopapillomas, with Ki67 and p53 expression, which is distinct from benign onychopapilloma cases [12].

Key Points

1. Onychopapilloma, a relatively common tumor of the nail bed and distal nail matrix, most commonly presents with longitudinal erythronychia with a distal subungual hyperkeratosis.
2. Dermoscopic features including distal subungual hyperkeratosis and splinter hemorrhages aid in making the diagnosis. Clinical follow-up is often recommended for asymptomatic cases, given its benign nature and low risk of malignancy.
3. Longitudinal excision with histopathology is essential for definitive diagnosis of patients with non-classic clinical findings or symptoms, and is needed to rule out malignant onychopapilloma, amelanotic melanoma, and SCC.

Funding Details   No funding was utilized for this study or manuscript.

Disclosure Statement   Authors ENA and SRL have no conflicts of interest to declare.

Financial Disclosures   Author SRL has served as a consultant for Eli Lilly, Ortho Dermatologics, Moberg Pharmaceuticals, and BelleTorus Corporation.

References

1. Halteh P, Magro C, Scher RK, Lipner SR. Onychopapilloma presenting as leukonychia: case report and review of the literature. Skin Appendage Disord. 2017;2(3–4):89–91. https://doi.org/10.1159/000448105. Epub 2017/02/25. PubMed PMID: 28232912; PMCID: PMC5264471
2. Baran R, Perrin C. Longitudinal erythronychia with distal subungual keratosis: onychopapilloma of the nail bed and Bowen's disease. Br J Dermatol. 2000;143(1):132–5. https://doi.org/10.1046/j.1365-2133.2000.03602.x. Epub 2000/07/25
3. Mattioli MA, Aromolo IF, Spigariolo CB, Marzano AV, Nazzaro G. Sonographic features of onychopapilloma: a single center retrospective observational study. J Clin Med. 2023;12(5) https://doi.org/10.3390/jcm12051795. Epub 2023/03/12. PubMed PMID: 36902582; PMCID: PMC10003362.
4. Yun JSW, Howard A, Prakash S, Kern JS. Clinical and histopathological features of onychopapilloma in an Australian setting: a case series of 50 patients. Australas J Dermatol. 2022;63(4):e350–e5. https://doi.org/10.1111/ajd.13900. Epub 2022/07/30. PubMed PMID: 35904503; PMCID: PMC9796568
5. Tosti A, Schneider SL, Ramirez-Quizon MN, Zaiac M, Miteva M. Clinical, dermoscopic, and pathologic features of onychopapilloma: a review of 47 cases. J Am Acad Dermatol. 2016;74(3):521–6. https://doi.org/10.1016/j.jaad.2015.08.053. Epub 2015/11/01
6. Delvaux C, Richert B, Lecerf P, André J. Onychopapillomas: a 68-case series to determine best surgical procedure and histologic sectioning. J Eur Acad Dermatol Venereol. 2018;32(11):2025–30. https://doi.org/10.1111/jdv.15037. Epub 2018/05/08
7. Conway J, Magro CM, Lipner SR. Expanding the differential diagnosis of the painful nail: a case of an onychopapilloma with neuroma. Case Rep Dermatol. 2024;16(1):88–93. https://doi.org/10.1159/000538087. Epub 20240328. PubMed PMID: 38550795; PMCID: PMC10978039

8. Kim TR, Bae KN, Son JH, Shin K, Kim HS, Ko HC, Kim BS, Kim MB. Onychopapilloma: its clinical, dermoscopic and pathologic features. J Eur Acad Dermatol Venereol. 2022;36(11):2235–40. https://doi.org/10.1111/jdv.18461. Epub 2022/07/24

9. Jellinek NJ, Lipner SR. Longitudinal erythronychia: retrospective single-center study evaluating differential diagnosis and the likelihood of malignancy. Dermatologic Surg. 2016;42(3):310–9. https://doi.org/10.1097/dss.0000000000000594.

10. Haynes D, Haneke E, Rubin AI. Clinical, onychoscopic, nail clipping, and histopathological findings of malignant onychopapilloma. J Cutan Pathol. 2024. Epub 20240402; https://doi.org/10.1111/cup.14620.

11. Haneke E, Iorizzo M, Gabutti M, Beltraminelli H. Malignant onychopapilloma. J Cutan Pathol. 2021;48(1):174–9. https://doi.org/10.1111/cup.13904. Epub 20201109

12. André J, Ewbank A, Moulonguet I, Richert B. Three atypical/malignant onychopapillomas in a 52-case series with immunohistochemical study. J Cutan Pathol. 2024;51(3):239–45. https://doi.org/10.1111/cup.14558. Epub 20231106

Chapter 18
White Nails in a Man with Hepatic Cirrhosis

Noreen Khan (iD) **and Julie Mervak** (iD)

Abstract Apparent leukonychia, a nail bed abnormality, can be differentiated from true leukonychia, a nail plate abnormality, by applying pressure to the nail plate and observing that leukonychia dissipates. Terry's nails (total apparent leukonychia) are a common finding in patients with hepatic cirrhosis but can be seen in other systemic illnesses or normal aging. On clinical diagnosis of Terry's nails, evaluation for underlying associated systemic etiology should be considered, if not already known.

Keywords Leukonychia · Nail bed · White · Cirrhosis · Systemic disease

Clinical Case

A 64-year-old male with end stage liver disease secondary to alcohol abuse presented to the dermatology clinic and was noted on physical examination to have leukonychia of all 10 fingernails (Fig. 18.1). There was a 1 mm band of pink-brown color at the distal nail bed close to the nail plate free edge. The lunula was not visible. The white color faded with pressure applied to the nail plate. He denied associated pain or difficulty trimming his nails.

N. Khan · J. Mervak (✉)
University of Michigan Medical School (NK), University of Michigan Department of Dermatology – Michigan Medicine (JM), Ann Arbor, MI, USA
e-mail: noreenk@med.umich.edu; jheringh@med.umich.edu

Fig. 18.1 Diffuse
leukonychia of the
fingernails with 1 mm
pink-brown band at the
distal nail bed

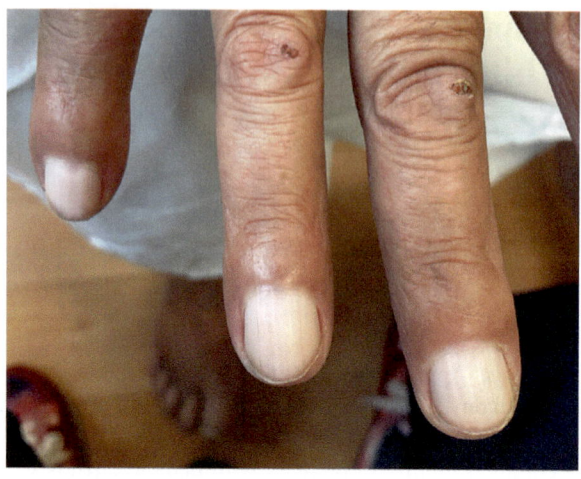

Based on the Case Description and the Photographs, What Is Your Diagnosis?

1. Lindsay's nails (partial apparent leukonychia)
2. Terry's nails (total apparent leukonychia)
3. True leukonychia
4. Muehrcke's lines (transverse apparent leukonychia)

Diagnosis

Terry's nails (total apparent leukonychia)

Discussion

In 1954, physician Richard Terry noted abnormal white nails in 82% of patients with hepatic cirrhosis, the majority due to alcohol use [1]. This phenomenon of total apparent leukonychia in patients thus has the eponym "Terry's nails," and describes the appearance of uniform, symmetric white nail beds with no visible lunula and greater than 80% of the nail involved [2]. Apparent leukonychia, in contrast to true leukonychia, represents abnormality of the nail bed and not the nail plate, and the white color will fade when pressure is applied. There is a thin distal band of normal pink to pink-brown color, 0.5 mm to 3 mm wide [3]. This is thought to represent a prominent onychodermal band and pathology at this distal site shows telangiectasias [2, 3]. The pink-brown color seen in some patients with Terry's nails has not correlated well on histology as there is no increase in melanin or hemosiderin [3]. It is speculated that apparent leukonychia represents a change in nail bed vascularity due to overgrowth of connective tissue [4], however there is still some question surrounding the pathophysiology.

Terry's nails are thought to be a reliable physical examination finding in patients with cirrhosis and early autoimmune hepatitis [5, 6], but can also be a sign of other systemic diseases including chronic renal failure, congestive heart failure, and adult-onset diabetes [2]. These nail changes can also be seen in normal aging without associated systemic disease. It has been hypothesized that cirrhosis and these other systemic diseases "age the nail" at an accelerated rate [3].

The differential diagnosis for Terry's nails includes Lindsay's nails (also known as half-and-half nails or partial apparent leukonychia), true leukonychia, and Muehrcke's lines (transverse apparent leukonychia), all of which present with white discoloration of the nail.

Lindsay's nails describe leukonychia which resolves with pressure, however the leukonychia involves less than 80% of the nail bed with the remaining distal red-brown color. This is most commonly seen in patients with chronic renal disease, particularly those requiring hemodialysis. This has also been reported in hepatic cirrhosis, Crohn's disease, pellagra, or healthy individuals [2].

True leukonychia represents an abnormality of the nail plate, and not the nail bed. This is seen in punctate, transverse, longitudinal or rarely total leukonychia patterns. This does not improve with pressure applied to the nail plate. Total true leukonychia of isolated digits can be seen in the setting of neurovascular insufficiency. True leukonychia of all digits is uncommon and seen in rare genetic disorders [2].

Muehrcke's lines (transverse apparent leukonychia) are transverse bands of leukonychia which improve with pressure. This does not involve the entire nail bed as would be the case with Terry's nails. Hypoalbuminemia is the most common association and once this is corrected the nail changes also resolve [7].

Terry's nails are a clinical diagnosis without need for histology. Prompt evaluation for underlying liver disease should be considered if this diagnosis is not already established. There is no consensus on resolution of Terry's nails after liver transplantation as this has been reported to improve in some individuals and persist in others [8, 9].

Key Points

- Apparent leukonychia, a nail bed abnormality, can be differentiated from true leukonychia, a nail plate abnormality, by applying pressure to the nail plate to observe if the leukonychia fades.
- Terry's nails (total apparent leukonychia) are a common finding in patients with hepatic cirrhosis but can be seen in other systemic illnesses or normal aging.
- There is no treatment specifically for Terry's nails and reports of resolution after liver transplantation are mixed.

References

1. Terry R. White nails in hepatic cirrhosis. Lancet. 1954;266(6815):757–9. https://doi.org/10.1016/s0140-6736(54)92717-8.
2. Iorizzo M, Starace M, Pasch MC. Leukonychia: what can white nails tell us? Am J Clin Dermatol. 2022;23(2):177–93. https://doi.org/10.1007/s40257-022-00671-6.
3. Holzberg M, Walker HK. Terry's nails: revised definition and new correlations. Lancet. 1984;8382:896–9. https://doi.org/10.1016/s0140-6736(84)91351-5.
4. Witkowska AB, Jasterzbski TJ, Schwartz RA. Terry's nails: a sign of systemic disease. Indian J Dermatol. 2017;62(3):309–11. https://doi.org/10.4103/ijd.IJD_98_17.
5. Udell JA, Wang CS, Tinmouth J, FitzGerald JM, Ayas NT, Simel DL, et al. Does this patient with liver disease have cirrhosis? JAMA. 2012;307(8):832–42. https://doi.org/10.1001/jama.2012.186.
6. Navarro-Trivino FJ, Linares-Gonzalez L, Rodenas-Herranz T. Terry's nails as the first clinical sign of autoimmune hepatitis. Rev Clin Esp. 2020;220(9):603–4. https://doi.org/10.1016/j.rce.2019.02.009.
7. Williams V, Jayashree M. Muehrcke's lines in an infant. J Pediatr. 2017;189:234. https://doi.org/10.1016/j.jpeds.2017.05.039.
8. Shrimal A, Gupte AA. Nail changes in cirrhosis and reversal after adult & pediatric liver transplantation. J Clin Exp Hepatol. 2020;10(5):531–2. https://doi.org/10.1016/j.jceh.2020.04.005.
9. Sarac G, Ozcan KN, Baskiran A, Cenk H, Sarac M, Sener S, Yilmaz S. Dermatological signs in liver transplant patients. J Cosmet Dermatol. 2021;20(9):2969–74. https://doi.org/10.1111/jocd.13944.

Chapter 19
Chroma Quest: A Tale of Melanonychia Mayhem

Marita Yaghi and Brian W Morrison

Abstract Exogenous chromonychia is a rare but important diagnostic consideration in cases of nail pigmentation. We present a 69-year-old male with progressive, asymptomatic grey discoloration affecting all fingernails for over 2 years. Extensive workup, including histopathology and fungal studies, was negative for infectious or melanocytic pathology. Detailed history revealed long-term use of a grey-reducing hair coloring shampoo, containing 1,2,4-Trihydroxybenzene (1,2,4-THB), a compound linked to pigmentary changes. Following discontinuation of the shampoo, the nail discoloration nearly resolved. This case underscores the significance of thorough exposure history in evaluating melanonychia and highlights an unusual but ubiquitous exogenous cause of nail pigmentation.

Keywords Melanonychia · Exogenous hyperpigmentation

Clinical Case

A 69-year-old male presented with a chief complaint of nail color changes affecting the fingernails that began more than 2 years ago. He described a pattern of waxing and waning nail alterations and denies any other symptoms. Previous work up with an outside healthcare provider, which included nail clippings sent for histopathology and fungal culture, showed no evidence of fungal infection.

Review of systems proved negative, notably for fingernail bleeding or ulceration as well as oral and throat symptoms. The patient reported a history of idiopathic familial polycythemia, for which he regularly donates blood every 3 months. He endorsed being concerned about the potential impact of his diagnosis on his nails. Current medications at the time included valsartan, atorvastatin, tamsulosin,

M. Yaghi · B. W Morrison (✉)
Dr. Phillip Frost Department of Dermatology and Cutaneous Surgery, University of Miami Miller School of Medicine, Miami, FL, USA
e-mail: Mxy537@med.miami.edu; Bmorrison@med.miami.edu

sildenafil and a testosterone pump, all of which he had been using long before the onset of his nail symptoms. Professionally, he works as an accountant with exclusive computer use and denied using any pen and paper which could lead to staining of his nails. When questioned about his habits, he noted the use of a coloring shampoo for his hair over the past few years did coincide with the onset of his nail changes.

On physical examination, diffuse grey total melanonychia affecting all 10 fingernails was noted (Fig. 19.1), proving resistant to removal with acetone or alcohol application. Dermoscopy revealed numerous grey granules (Figs. 19.2 and 19.3). A full-body skin exam, including toenail examination, revealed no additional abnormalities.

Nail clippings were collected for histopathological examination. Microscopic examination revealed compact hyperkeratosis with focal parakeratosis, along with an intraepithelial, predominantly neutrophilic, infiltrate. No melanin or iron were detected with Fontana-Mason Special staining and Prussian Blue special staining respectively.

Fig. 19.1 Melanonychia affecting all 10 fingernails

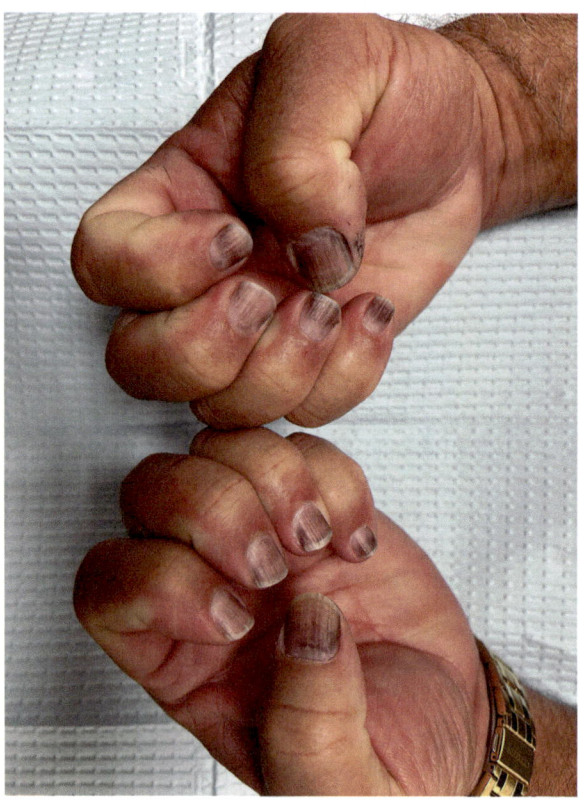

Fig. 19.2 Dermoscopic image of the left thumb showing diffuse grey granules

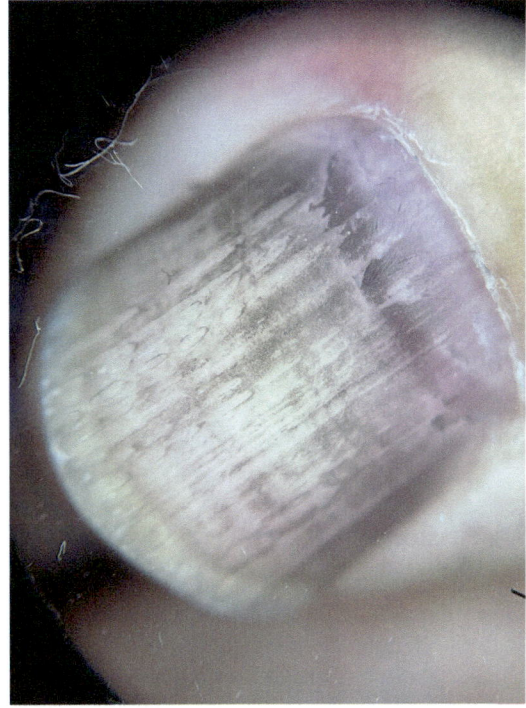

Fig. 19.3 Dermoscopic image of the left 5th digit showing diffuse grey granules with pronounced concentration on the distal aspect of the nail unit

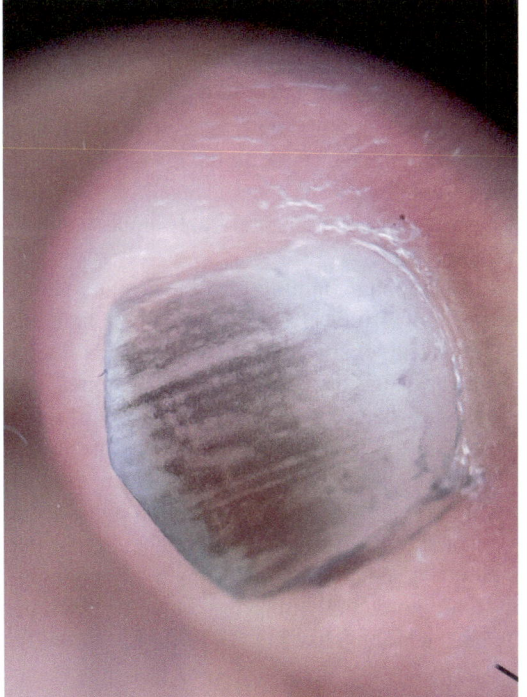

Based on the Case Description and the Photographs, What Is Your Diagnosis?

A. Candidal onychomycosis
B. Shampoo-induced melanonychia
C. Drug-induced nail melanonychia
D. Nail hyperpigmentation secondary to polycythemia
E. 10-digit subungual melanoma

Diagnosis

Shampoo-induced melanonychia

Discussion

Given the clinical presentation and course of the patient's manifestations, along with the dermatopathological findings, a diagnosis of shampoo-induced melano-nychia, likely a result of hair colorants, was rendered. Therefore, the patient was reassured and instructed to discontinue the use of the shampoo until his follow-up appointment 3 months later, at which point the melanonychia had nearly cleared.

Ungual dyschromia, or chromonychia, refers to the discoloration of the nail plate or subungual nail bed. Discoloration of the normally transparent nail can stem from a variety of factors affecting the nail plate or the underlying nail bed [1]. Alterations in nail color can arise from external sources such as trauma, infection, or occupa-tional exposure, or from the overproduction or accumulation of endogenously derived pigments. Determining the anatomical source of the chromonychia requires the assessment of the specific anatomical pattern of involvement through a detailed physical examination, preferably under natural light with the hands in a relaxed position [2].

Predominant staining of the nail plate along the proximal fold can indicate an exogenous origin [1, 2]. Rarely, pigmentation following the shape of the lunula signifies an overproduction or storage of endogenous pigment [2]. Successful removal of the discoloration with acetone suggests a topical agent as the culprit. Fading of the color with slight pressure to the nail suggests alterations in nail bed vasculature, while persistence of the discoloration indicates an abnormality lying within the nail plate. In cases where the dyschromia makes it hard to assess struc-tural nail changes, transillumination against the finger pulp may help identify the presence of markings, pitting, thickening, or detachment of the nail plate from the nail bed when present, distorting the normal nail plate's uniform reddish glow [2].

Chromonychia with grey, brown or black pigmentation is specifically referred to as melanonychia [1]. It is further broadly categorized as caused by either melanocyte activation or and underlying melanocytic neoplasm. Mono- and poly-dactylous longitudinal melanonychia due to melanocyte activation is common, especially in Fitzpatrick skin phototypes V and VI, affecting approximately 15–20% of Asians and up to 70% of African-Americans over 20 years old [3]. Total melanonychia, as seen in this patient, is much rarer, and may be a sign of a systemic underlying condition [4]. Our patient's asymptomatic presentation, coupled with the comprehensive and unremarkable examination of the skin and mucous membranes we performed showed no indication of a potential underlying disease. However, his regular use of a gray-reducing coloring shampoo and the sequential onset of his symptoms, we suspected that the shampoo could be a potential culprit agent.

To reinforce our diagnosis without resorting to invasive procedures like a nail biopsy, which would likely be non-diagnostic, we examined the shampoo's ingredient list and observed the presence of three distinct hair colorants: N, N-Bis(2-Hydroxyethyl)-p-Phenylenediamine Sulfate, p-aminophenol, and 1, 2, 4-Trihydroxybenzene (1,2,4-THB). 1,2,4-THB is also referred to hydroxyhydroquinone. The European Commission Scientific Committee on Consumer Safety (SCCS) has identified the presence of hydroquinone as an impurity in 1,2,4-THB -containing lots [5]. Hydroquinone is a common cause of exogenous ochronosis [6], or blue-black discoloration of the face, when used for long periods of time. Rare cases in the literature have reported nail discoloration secondary to hydroquinone, with the reported discoloration typically being orange brown in color [7–9]. As reports of this condition remain very scarce, it is possible that 1,2,4-THB or its metabolite, hydroquinone, are responsible for the total melanonychia seen in our patient.

In conclusion, a thorough clinical assessment is crucial to avoid unnecessary tests. Asking about environmental exposures and product use can provide vital clues. Our patient's diagnosis of shampoo-induced melanonychia was confirmed through careful examination and ingredient analysis, followed by resolution after discontinuing its use. Rare cases in the literature suggest a link between nail discoloration and hydroquinone, underscoring the need to consider uncommon causes. This highlights the value of non-invasive diagnostic methods and the complexities involved in diagnosing nail dyschromia.

Key Points

- Melanonychia, of black nail dyschromia, can originate from exogenous factors like trauma, infection or environmental exposure, or endogenous causes such as pigment overproduction or deposition.
- Accurate diagnosis requires a thorough clinical assessment, including detailed history-taking and physical examination of the nails, skin, and mucosal surfaces, to identify potential causal agents to the melanonychia and rule out any associated underlying condition.

- In assessing patients with melanonychia, it's imperative to explore both common and uncommon causes, including inquiries about grooming practices and professional exposures, among other factors, in an effort to avoid potential misdiagnoses and oversights.

References

1. Baran R, de Berker DAR, Holzberg M, Thomas L. Baran and Dawber's diseases of the nails and their management. 4th ed. Wiley-Blackwell; 2012.
2. Mendiratta V, Jain A. Nail dyschromias. Indian J Dermatol Venereol Leprol. 2011;77:652.
3. André J, Lateur N. Pigmented nail disorders. Dermatol Clin. 2006;24(3):329–39.
4. Jefferson J, Rich P. Melanonychia. Dermatol Res Pract. 2012;2012:952186.
5. Safety ECSCoC. Opinion on hair dye 1,2,4-trihydroxybenzene (1,2,4-THB), COLIPA n° A33 (CAS 533-73-3) 2019. https://health.ec.europa.eu/system/files/2021-08/sccs_o_222_0.pdf.
6. Bhattar PA, Zawar VP, Godse KV, Patil SP, Nadkarni NJ, Gautam MM. Exogenous ochronosis. Indian J Dermatol. 2015;60(6):537–43.
7. Glazer A, Sofen BD, Gallo ES. Nail discoloration after use of hydroquinone. JAAD Case Rep. 2016;2(1):57–8.
8. Mann R, Harman R. Nail staining due to hydroquinone skin-lightening creams. Br J Dermatol. 1983;108(3):363–5.
9. Parlak AH, Aydoğan İ, Kavak A. Discolouration of the fingernails from using hydroquinone skin-lightening cream. J Cosmet Dermatol. 2003;2(3-4):199–201.

Chapter 20
Nail Changes in a Chronic Male Smoker

Marita Yaghi and Brian W Morrison

Abstract This case report describes a 44-year-old Haitian male smoker who presented with rapid-onset progressive nail changes and hand eruptions, accompanied by a chronic six-month cough. Physical examination revealed extensive nail abnormalities including paronychia, anonychia, and nail bed hyperkeratosis, along with erythematous keratotic papules on the ears and hyperkeratotic plaques on the palm. While initial laboratory testing was unremarkable, chest imaging revealed a substantial mass in the left upper lobe suggestive of pulmonary malignancy. The patient was diagnosed with Acrokeratosis Paraneoplastica (Bazex syndrome), a rare paraneoplastic dermatosis that typically presents with psoriasiform eruptions and nail changes as early manifestations of underlying malignancy, particularly of the upper aerodigestive tract.

Keywords Bazex syndrome · Paraneoplastic syndrome · Nail dystrophy · Lung cancer

Clinical Case

A 44-year-old Haitian man presented to the clinic with rapid onset of progressively worsening nail changes and an eruption on his hands. He also reported a lingering chronic cough that had persisted for the past 6 months. The patient's past medical history was unremarkable, aside from a significant 40-pack-year history of cigarette smoking.

M. Yaghi · B. W Morrison (✉)
Dr. Phillip Frost Department of Dermatology and Cutaneous Surgery, University of Miami Miller School of Medicine, Miami, FL, USA
e-mail: Mxy537@med.miami.edu; Bmorrison@med.miami.edu

© The Author(s), under exclusive license to Springer Nature Switzerland AG 2025
A. Tosti et al. (eds.), *Clinical Cases in Nail Disorders*, Clinical Cases in Dermatology, https://doi.org/10.1007/978-3-031-88642-3_20

Physical examination of the fingers and toes exposed pronounced nail changes including paronychia with erythematous and edematous nail folds and hyponychium, anonychia and marked hyperkeratosis of the nail bed with some overlying yellow crust (Figs. 20.1 and 20.2). Further examination revealed multiple erythematous keratotic papules of the bilateral helices of the ear (Fig. 20.3) and a hyperkeratotic plaque on the left palm (Fig. 20.4). Hyperkeratotic, ulcerated papules on the proximal interphalangeal joints of the second and fifth digits of the left hand were also found (Fig. 20.1).

Laboratory testing revealed a complete blood count (CBC) and comprehensive metabolic panel (CMP) within the normal range. A non-reactive rapid plasma reagin (RPR) and negative human immunodeficiency virus (HIV) test results were also rendered. A chest X-ray unveiled a substantial mass located in the left upper lobe. Subsequent findings from a chest computed tomography (CT) scan showed extensive disease, suggestive of pulmonary malignancy.

Fig. 20.1 Erythema of the proximal and lateral nail folds, anonychia, nail bed hyperkeratosis and associated erosions extending beyond they hyponychium with some yellow crusting affecting all fingernails

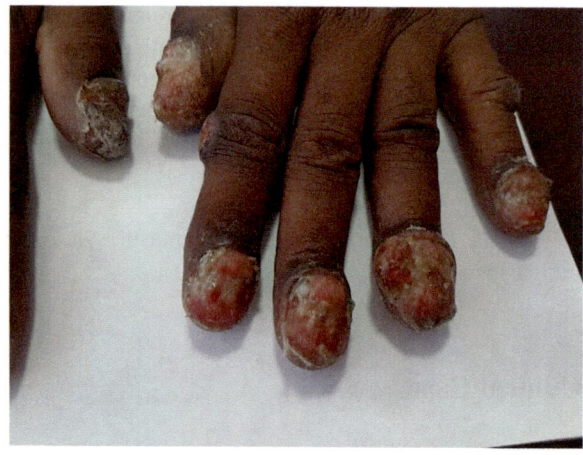

Fig. 20.2 Erythema and edema of the proximal and lateral nail folds, anonychia, nail bed hyperkeratosis and associated erosions extending beyond they hyponychium affecting the toenails

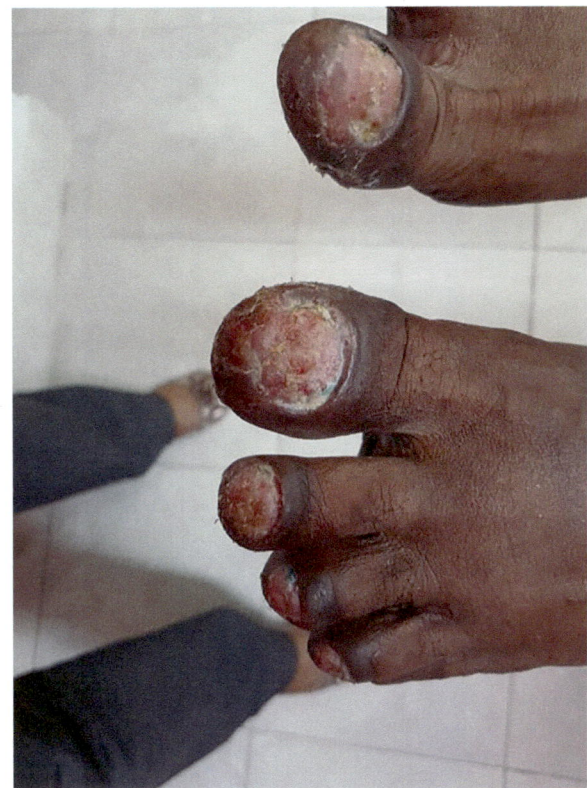

Fig. 20.3 Erythematous scaly papules affecting the helix of the left ear and some skin-colored papules on the left cheek

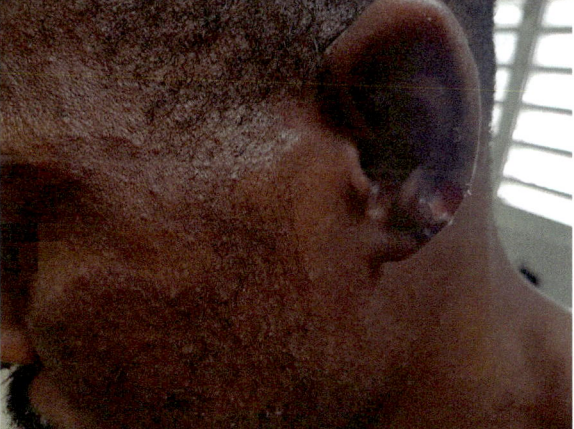

Fig. 20.4 Hyperlinear palm with a skin-colored hyperkeratotic plaque on the left palm

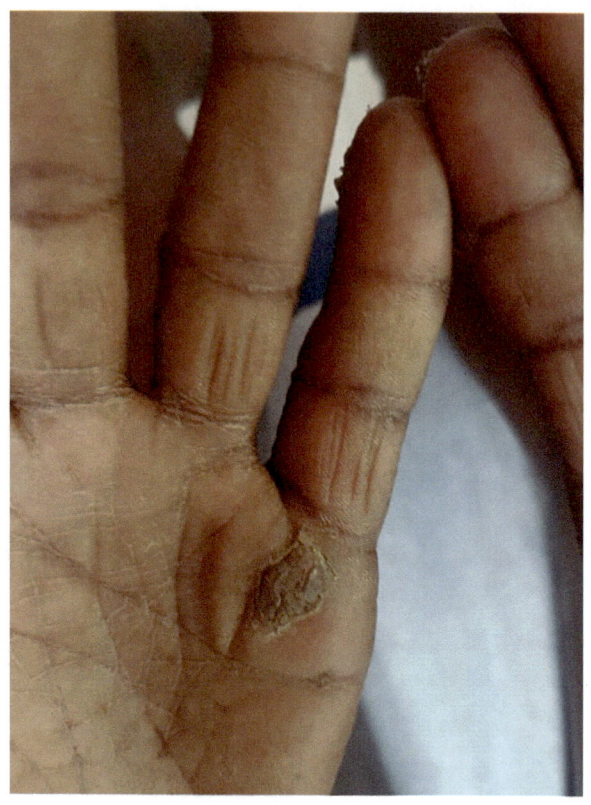

Based on the Case Description and the Photographs, What Is Your Diagnosis?

A. Acrodermatitis Continua of Hallopeau
B. Cutaneous T Cell Lymphoma
C. Acrokeratosis Paraneoplastic (Bazex Syndrome)
D. Hyperkeratotic rhagadiform hand and foot eczema
E. Epidermolysis bullosa acquisita

Diagnosis

Acrokeratosis Paraneoplastic (Bazex Syndrome)

Discussion

Acrokeratosis paraneoplastica (Bazex syndrome) is a rare paraneoplastic dermatosis characterized by psoriasiform eruption symmetrically affecting acral skin [1, 2]. First described in 1965, it has been linked to various internal malignancies, notably squamous cell carcinomas of the upper aerodigestive tract or metastatic disease to the cervical lymph nodes [1]. Cutaneous and ungual signs are typically the earliest manifestations, and therefore, high clinical suspicion should prompt an exhaustive investigation for potential malignancies [3].

Men are most affected by acrokeratosis paraneoplastica, in contrast with the female predominance observed with Acrodermatitis Continua of Hallopeau. In addition, the latter often harbors a geographic tongue, a finding that is a notably absent in Bazex Syndrome.

The typical clinical picture often involves symmetrical, psoriasiform papules and plaques on the nose, ear helices, digits, palms, and soles. Nail involvement has been documented in up to 75% of cases, with subungual hyperkeratosis, thickening or onychauxis, yellow/brown discoloration, onycholysis, longitudinal ridging and onychomadesis being the most prevalent observations [2]. Destruction, complete loss, fissuring, crumbling, and brittleness of the nail plate, along with paronychia with associated erythema, nail tenderness, clubbing, and cuticle loss have also been noted in certain instances [2], reflecting the diverse spectrum of nail-related manifestations associated with the condition.

According to Bazex et al., the disease develops in three stages, each with a distinctive clinical picture [1]. In stage 1, the ear lobes, ear helix, the tip of the nose, distal fingertips, or nails are primarily affected. Ungual involvement commonly reveals the presence of vesicles, subungual hyperkeratosis, or nail dystrophy. Stage 2 is characterized by frequent involvement of the palms and soles. Additionally, the condition progresses to affect areas such as the cheeks, forehead, elbows, thighs, and knees. Eruption spreading to the trunk is the hallmark of stage 3. It is crucial to note that the expansion of cutaneous manifestations does not necessarily indicate the growth of the underlying tumor.

A comprehensive workup is essential to identify the underlying malignancy. An otolaryngologic examination, chest X-ray or CT, CBC, CMP, erythrocyte sedimentation rate (ESR), and tumor markers such as carcinoembryonic antigen (CEA) should be first conducted to rule out malignancies affecting the pharynx, larynx or upper aerodigestive tract [4, 5]. Negative findings should prompt consideration for further investigations, including a gastrointestinal endoscopy, colonoscopy, testing for occult blood in stool, or additional markers such as CA-125 or prostate-specific antigen (PSA) [4, 5].

Treating the underlying malignancy is the mainstay of management. Improvement has been reported with the application of high-potency topical steroids, salicylic acid 10% in petrolatum, and the use of topical antifungals [5]. In more severe cases, systemic treatment with corticosteroids (prednisone 60 mg daily or dexamethasone 10 mg daily), retinoids (etretinate at 0.75-1 mg/kg/day or acitretin at 25 mg daily) or psoralen plus ultraviolet A (PUVA) therapy have been beneficial [5, 6]. Notably, cutaneous and ungual manifestations may resolve with tumor remission [3, 5], and their reappearance should be regarded as a potential sign of relapse [3, 5], prompting further attention and assessment.

Key Points

- Bazex Syndrome is a rare, acral paraneoplastic dermatosis characterized by symmetrical, psoriasiform eruption and a wide range of nail manifestations.
- Nail involvement, observed in 75% of cases, encompasses presents a spectrum of abnormalities, spanning subungual hyperkeratosis and onycholysis, alongside distinctive features like thickening, discoloration, longitudinal ridging, and onychomadesis.
- Cutaneous and ungual manifestations are often the initial manifestations and should prompt an exhaustive malignancy work-up, first focused on the upper aerodigestive tract.
- Nail abnormalities play a crucial role in the clinical presentation of Bazex syndrome, emphasizing the significance of recognizing and understanding these ungual signs for accurate diagnosis and effective management.

References

1. Bazex A, Griffiths A. Acrokeratosis paraneoplastica—a new cutaneous marker of malignancy. Br. J. Dermatol. 1980;103(3):301–6.
2. Roy B, Lipner SR. A review of nail changes in acrokeratosis paraneoplastica (Bazex syndrome). Skin Appendage Disord. 2021;7(3):163–72.
3. Arnal C, Richert B. Nail disorders to be kept in mind. Hand Surg Rehabil. 2024:101640.
4. Abreu Velez AM, Howard MS. Diagnosis and treatment of cutaneous paraneoplastic disorders. Dermatol Ther. 2010;23(6):662–75.
5. Räßler F, Goetze S, Elsner P. Acrokeratosis paraneoplastica (Bazex syndrome)–a systematic review on risk factors, diagnosis, prognosis and management. J Eur Acad Dermatol Venereol. 2017;31(7):1119–36.
6. Conde-Montero E, Baniandrés-Rodríguez O, Horcajada-Reales C, Parra-Blanco V, Suárez-Fernández R. Paraneoplastic acrokeratosis (Bazex syndrome): unusual association with in situ follicular lymphoma and response to acitretin. Cutis. 2017;100(2):E3–5.

Chapter 21
A Case of Severe Onychogryphosis

Lawrence Chukwudi Nwabudike (ID)

Abstract Onychogryphosis, is a nail disorder characterised by thickening and yellowish brown discoloration. It is most commonly acquired, but may also be congenital or associated with some genodermatoses.

A case of a 45-year old female with nail deformity consequent upon an 8-year history of not cutting her nails and rarely leaving home. Examination revealed thickened, brown, twisted toenails with transverse ridges along their length. The great toenails were most severely affected, with the right measuring approximately 7 cm. She was diagnosed with onychogryphosis, the nails were cut and she was recommended psychiatric care, but became lost to followup.

Onychogryphosis is a common nail disorder, which may be congenital or acquired. The congenital form is rarer and is often autosomal dominant. The therapy may be conservative or surgical.

In this chapter a case of onychogryphosis is presented with a review of the disorder.

Keywords Onychogryphosis · Ram's horn nails · Nail disease · Pachyonychia congenita · Onychomycosis

Introduction

Onychogryphosis, also known as ram's horn nails, is a disorder characterized by excessive and abnormal growth of the nails, with thickening and yellowish-brown discoloration. It is most commonly acquired, but onychogryphosis of congenital origin as well as in connection with some genodermatoses has been described.

A case of severe onychogryphosis involving both feet is presented.

L. C. Nwabudike (✉)
N. Paulescu National Institute of Diabetes, Bucharest, Romania

N. Paulescu National Institute of Diabetes, Bucharest, Dermatology, Bucharest, Romania

© The Author(s), under exclusive license to Springer Nature Switzerland AG 2025
A. Tosti et al. (eds.), *Clinical Cases in Nail Disorders*, Clinical Cases in Dermatology, https://doi.org/10.1007/978-3-031-88642-3_21

123

Fig. 21.1 Brown, thickened and twisted, overgrown toenails resembling ram horns

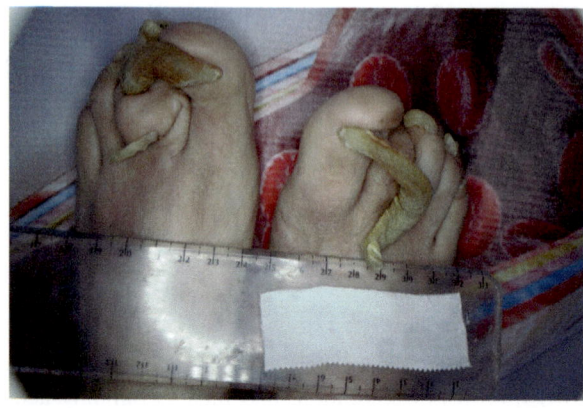

The Case

A 45-year old female presented with a history of persistent nail deformity. The patient's mother stated that she hardly left the house and had not cut her nails in about 8 years(!). No history of psychiatric disorder could be elucidated.

Examination revealed a healthy-looking female with brown, thickened, twisted toenails (Fig. 21.1). Transverse ridges along the length of the nails were also observed. All toenails with the exception of the left fifth toenail were affected. Those of the large toes bilaterally were most severely affected, with the right large toenail measuring approximately 7 cm. There was no tenderness to palpation.

A diagnosis of severe toenail onychogryphosis was made, based on the clinical features of the disorder.

Differential Diagnosis

- Congenital malalignment of the toenails—usually presents at birth or shortly thereafter. It is thought to be autosomal dominant. This was not the case with this patient.
- Pachyonychia congenita—caused by an autosomal dominant mutation of genes and usually affects the fingers.
- Onychomycosis—very common, but does not present with ram's horn nails seen in this patient.

The nails were cut under local anesthesia and dressed. The patient returned the following day for a followup visit (Figs. 21.2a, b). She was recommended specialist (psychiatric) care and became lost to followup.

Fig. 21.2 (**a**, **b**) Toenails cut to normal size and shape

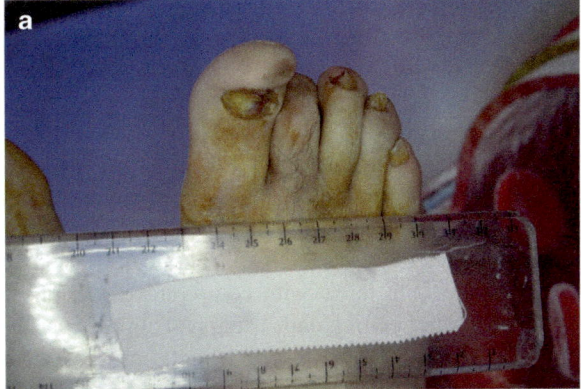

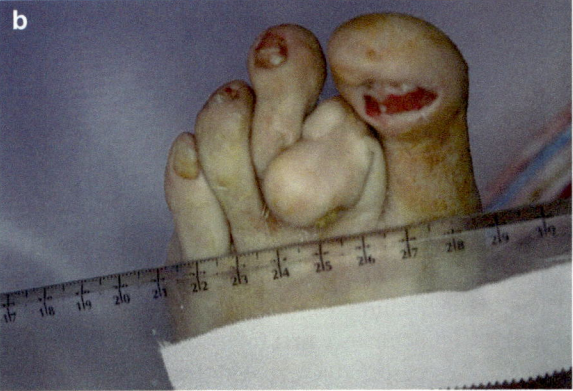

Discussion

Onychogryphosis is a nail disorder caused by disordered nail growth [1]. It is characterized by nail opacity, thickening, hyperkeratosis, increased curvature and elongation [2]. Nail thickening is the initial manifestation of onychogryphosis, followed by other changes that give the classic "ram's horn" or "oyster shape" appearance [3], making the early stages difficult to diagnose.

The prevalence appears greater in the elderly [3], varying between 11.2–38% [3, 4].

The cause is not known, but it is associated with advanced age, self-neglect, dementia, poor hygiene, ichthyosis, psoriasis, smallpox and syphilis [2, 3].

Onychogryphosis can be congenital or acquired [2, 3]. Both toe- and fingernails can be affected. The *congenital* form is rare and thought to be autosomal dominant [2, 3]. It may be associated with other genetic disorders such as pachyonychia congenita and Haim-Munk syndrome [2]. Some apparently idiopathic forms have been described. One case was of a 2-year old child who was reported to have had anonychia at birth, followed by onychogryphosis [5]. There was no family history of onychogryphosis. Another case was of a 45-year old male, with onychogryphosis of the left fifth finger since birth [6]. There was no family history recorded in this case either. The appearance of the nail caused the authors to think of the Tower of Pisa and they therefore described it as "leaning tower nail" [6]. The *acquired* form is associated with factors, such as neglect, poor hygiene, homelessness, ichthyosis, psoriasis, syphilis, smallpox, peripheral vascular disease and onychomycosis, amongst others [2, 3].

Potential complications of this disorder may include secondary onychomycosis, paronychia and foot ulcers resulting from trauma on other toes caused by the pathological nail; subungual gangrene may also occur.

Therapy may be conservative or surgical. Conservative methods are preferred in the elderly and in those with compromised peripheral vasculature. Conservative therapy includes cutting nails using nail clippers or a burr [2]. Finding shoes that fit the patient are indicated as prophylactic measures. Surgical therapy includes nail avulsion with or without matricectomy.

This case was successfully treated conservatively, but was subsequently lost to control.

Conclusions

Onychogryphosis is a common disorder and may be congenital or acquired. The congenital form is most often autosomal dominant or a component of certain syndromes. The acquired form is associated with neglect, advanced age, neurological disorders, inflammatory and infectious disorders. Therapy may be conservative or surgical. We presented a case with longstanding (8 years) acquired onychogryphosis, probably secondary to neglect, who underwent successful conservative therapy.

Key Points

1. Onychogryphosis is a common disorder.
2. It may be congenital or acquired. The congenital form is rare.
3. Diagnosis is clinical, based on the classic "ram's horn" appearance of the nails.
4. Therapy may be conservative or surgical.

References

1. Nakao A. Onychogryphosis https://dermnetnz.org/topics/onychogryphosis, 2019. Accessed 15 May 2024.
2. Ko D, Lipner SR. Onychogryphosis: case report and review of the literature. Skin Appendage Disord. 2018;4(4):326–30. https://doi.org/10.1159/000485854.
3. Chang P, Meaux T. Onychogryphosis: a report of ten cases. Skinmed. 2015;13(5):355–9. PMID: 26790505.

4. Ebrahim SB, Sainsbury R, Watson S. Foot problems of the elderly: a hospital survey. Br Med J (Clin Res Ed). 1981;283(6297):949–50. https://doi.org/10.1136/bmj.283.6297.949.
5. Sequeira JH. Case of congenital onychogryphosis. Proc R Soc Med. 1923;16(Dermatol Sect):92.
6. Nath AK, Udayashankar C. Congenital onychogryphosis: leaning tower nail. Dermatol Online J. 2011;17(11):9.

Chapter 22
A Case of Transverse White Nail Plate Bands

Elżbieta Wójtowicz and Paweł Pietkiewicz (iD)

Abstract White nails, a common form of nail discoloration, can be classified into three primary types: true leukonychia, apparent leukonychia, and pseudoleukonychia, each with distinct etiologies and clinical presentations. Diagnosis relies on medical assessment, detailed patient history, and physical examination, with onychoscopy aiding differentiation between types. Management focuses on addressing underlying causes and avoiding nail trauma. This comprehensive approach ensures effective treatment and recovery while preventing recurrence.

Here, we report the case of a 54-year-old female tailor who presented with transverse white bands involving multiple fingernails.

Keywords Transverse leukonychia · White nails · True leukonychia · Occupational nail trauma · Onychoscopy

Clinical Case

A 54-year-old female, tailor by occupation, presented at the dermatology outpatient clinic with transverse white bands and brittle nails that were present for many months. Multiple fingernails were affected (Fig. 22.1). Her medical history in regard to drug intake, diseases and allergies was non-contributory. She had no history of psoriasis. The white bands did not fade under compression. The patient underwent the following diagnostic tests: complete blood count, blood smear, sedimentation rate, CRP, aminotransferases, serum albumin, serum creatinine, serum lead and arsenic levels were within the normal limits. Electrocardiography, chest X-ray, and abdominal ultrasonography revealed no pathology.

E. Wójtowicz (✉)
Centrum Leczenia Nowotworów Skóry i Czerniaka, 5 Wojskowy Szpital Kliniczny z Polikliniką w Krakowie, Kraków, Poland

P. Pietkiewicz
Centrum Medyczne Zwierzyniecka, Poznań, Poland

© The Author(s), under exclusive license to Springer Nature Switzerland AG 2025
A. Tosti et al. (eds.), *Clinical Cases in Nail Disorders*, Clinical Cases in Dermatology, https://doi.org/10.1007/978-3-031-88642-3_22

Fig. 22.1 Multiple
fingernails affected with
transverse white lines
(better seen in box)

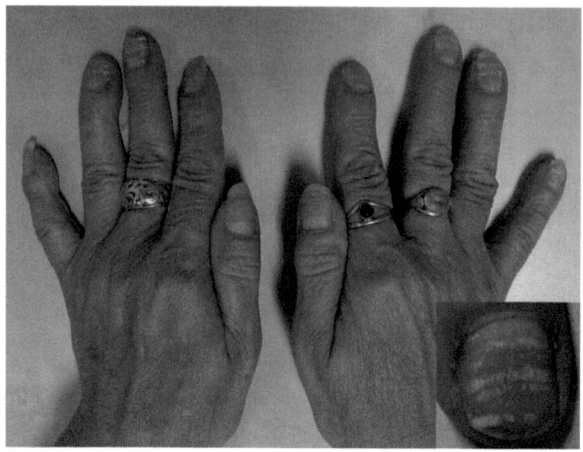

Based on the Case Description and the Photographs, What Is Your Diagnosis?

1. Trauma-induced transverse true leukonychia (Mees' lines)
2. Apparent transverse leukonychia (Muehrcke's lines)
3. White superficial onychomycosis
4. Nail psoriasis

Diagnosis

Trauma-induced transverse true leukonychia (Mees' lines)

Discussion

White nails are a prevalent form of nail dyschromia, which can be categorized into three primary types: true leukonychia, stemming from abnormalities in the nail matrix; apparent leukonychia, involving subungual tissue; and pseudo-leukonychia, caused by external factors (e.g. cosmetics or fungal infections). All variants may manifest as white transverse lines across the fingernails and/or toenails [1].

The white colour of the nail plates in true transverse leukonychia results from a structural alteration within the nail material itself, caused by abnormal keratinization of the distal matrix. Clinically, it presents as non-blanching transverse white bands parallel to the lunula, and moving distally with the nail growth. Repeated insult to the distal nail matrix can produce multiple parallel transverse white lines.

Transverse true leukonychia was first described by Rudolf A. Mees in 1919 in patients experiencing arsenic intoxication. Since that time many other causes of the transverse true leukonychia have been reported. Subsequent reports have identified various causes, including traumatic, over-zealous manicures or pedicures, cryotherapy of the warts of the proximal nail fold, repetitive trauma to the toenail's free edge, and direct occupational or recreational contact with a range of exogenous irritant. Systemic conditions should be considered when multiple transverse lines appear in both fingernails and toenails. Causes of true transverse leukonychia include chemotherapeutics (e.g. cyclosporin, cytostatics), heavy metal poisoning (thallium, strontium, arsenic), hematologic disorders (acute myeloid leukaemia, Hodgkin lymphoma), infectious diseases (tuberculosis, COVID, leprosy, malaria, herpes zoster), dermatologic conditions (psoriasis, erythema multiforme) and other systemic diseases (e.g. SLE), as well as nutritional deficiencies [2, 3].

Transverse white lines caused by apparent leukonychia are called Muehrcke's lines after Robert C. Muehrcke who first reported the finding in 1956 in patients with severe hypoalbuminemia. Muehrcke's lines are paired, narrowed pale lines originating from vascular congestion in the nail bed. They fade with compression and do not advance with the nail growth. Muehrcke's lines often develop in the second, third, and fourth fingernails, but rarely involve the thumbnail. Currently, Muehrcke lines are considered indicative of a range of systemic disorders presenting with or without hypoalbuminemia, including kidney and liver diseases, rheumatoid arthritis or in heart transplants. Various culprit drugs have been reported including systemic retinoids and cytostatics [4].

Pseudoleukonychia caused by nail cosmetics or manicure procedures is a common finding. The process of nail polish binding to, and subsequently being removed from the nail plate may lead to keratin degranulation. The clinical presentation encompasses usually white, scally nail plate macules and patches, yet in some instances the scaling areas may be arranged in a linear fashion forming white transverse bands [5]. Superficial white onychomycosis (*leukonychia trichophytica*) can also rarely present as transverse white bands on the toenails and less frequently fingernails. These white bands are usually randomly distributed along the surface of the nail plate and involve several neighbouring nail plates [2].

In majority of cases, the diagnosis of transverse leukonychia is clinical as detailed history (including lesions' evolution, personal medical and family history, occupation and hobbies) and physical examination are usually sufficient to identify a culprit factor [6]. It is of utmost importance to examine not only the nail apparatus areas being the main complain of the patient but perform full physical examination, in order not to overlook, and/or misinterpret other symptoms [6]. If fingernails are affected exclusively, it is crucial to inquire about nail care practices. When both fingernails and toenails are involved, detailed review of medications and supplements administered, as well as clinical/laboratory tests are recommended to rule out toxic or systemic aetiology. Onychoscopy is an auxiliary examination, increasing diagnostic confidence and facilitating the differential diagnosis. When examining the nails with white bands it is advisable to begin with a non-contact mode, as this method allows better visualization of scales of keratin granulation in pseudoleukonychia. Following this, a contact polarized dermatoscopy with interface medium (optimally a thick silicone gel) should be performed. The differentiation between apparent leukonychia (where Muehrcke's lines fade) and true leukonychia (where there is no fading) can be achieved by applying pressure, e.g. with a dermatoscope contact plate [2].

The management of the transverse leukonychia ultimately depends on the presence and addressing any underlying cause. Avoiding traumatic nail care procedures, such as excessive use of nail polish or excessive mechanical force with false nail application/removal, is vital for full and lasting recovery [1–3].

Key Points

- Vast range of conditions can contribute to the formation of transverse white nail bands, from simple manicure habits to life-threatening systemic intoxication, necessitating obtaining a meticulous assessment in each case.
- History and physical examination is often sufficient for making the diagnosis.
- Treatment ultimately depends on any underlying cause.
- Abstaining from traumatic manicure procedures will prevent recurrence of transverse white nail bands.

References

1. Baran R, Drawber RPR, editors. Diseases of the nails and their management. 2nd ed. Oxford: Blackwell Scientific Publications; 1994.
2. Iorizzo M, Starace M, Pasch MC. Leukonychia: what can white nails tell us? Am J Clin Dermatol. 2022;23(2):177–93. https://doi.org/10.1007/s40257-022-00671-6. Epub 2022 Feb 2. PMID: 35112320; PMCID: PMC8809498.
3. Piraccini BM, editor. Nail disorders: a practical guide to diagnosis and management. Milan: Springer; 2014.
4. Ramachandran V, Sapra A. Muehrcke lines of the fingernails. [Updated 2023 Jul 31]. In: StatPearls [Internet]. Treasure Island (FL): StatPearls Publishing; 2024 Jan-. Available from: https://www.ncbi.nlm.nih.gov/books/NBK559136.
5. Rieder EA, Tosti A. Cosmetically induced disorders of the nail with update on contemporary nail manicures. J Clin Aesthet Dermatol. 2016;9(4):39–44. Epub 2016 Apr 1. PMID: 27462387; PMCID: PMC4898583.
6. Pietkiewicz P, Bowszyc-Dmochowska M, Gornowicz-Porowska J, Dmochowski M. Involvement of nail apparatus in pemphigus vulgaris in ethnic poles is infrequent. Front Med (Lausanne). 2018;14(5):227. https://doi.org/10.3389/fmed.2018.00227. PMID: 30155468; PMCID: PMC6102408.

Chapter 23
Bilateral Median Transverse Ridging of the Thumb Nails in a Young Man

Paweł Pietkiewicz ⓘ**, Norbert Kiss** ⓘ**, and Magdalena Żychowska** ⓘ

Abstract A 50-year-old physical worker presented at the dermatology outpatient clinic with bilateral irregular transverse ridging of his thumbnails. There was no subungual hyperkeratosis and both the proximal nail fold and distal free edge of the nail plate were unaffected. Dermatoscopic examination revealed irregular transverse indentations in the dorsal aspect of the nail plate, forming a median canal.

Keywords Tic-habit deformity · Median canaliform dystrophy of Heller · Onychoscopy

Clinical Case

A 30-year-old physical worker presented at the dermatology outpatient clinic with bilateral changes of his thumbnails present for many years (Fig. 23.1). He reported transient amelioration of the lesions during administration of oral antibiotics. There was no history of psoriasis or other dermatological condition in the family, and the patient's medical history was non-contributory. Both nail plates featured irregular transverse ridging (variable in distance and width), yet were normal in color. There was no subungual hyperkeratosis and both the proximal nail fold and distal free edge of the nail plate were unaffected. No other nail changes were observed.

P. Pietkiewicz (✉)
Centrum Medyczne Zwierzyniecka, Poznań, Poland

N. Kiss
Department of Dermatology, Venereology and Dermatooncology, Semmelweis University, Budapest, Hungary
e-mail: kiss.norbert@med.semmelweis-univ.hu

M. Żychowska
Department of Dermatology, Institute of Medical Sciences, Medical College of Rzeszów University, Rzeszów, Poland

133

A. Tosti et al. (eds.), *Clinical Cases in Nail Disorders*, Clinical Cases in Dermatology, https://doi.org/10.1007/978-3-031-88642-3_23

Fig. 23.1 Transverse ridges radiating from a paramedian canal of a thumb nail in a 30-years old man

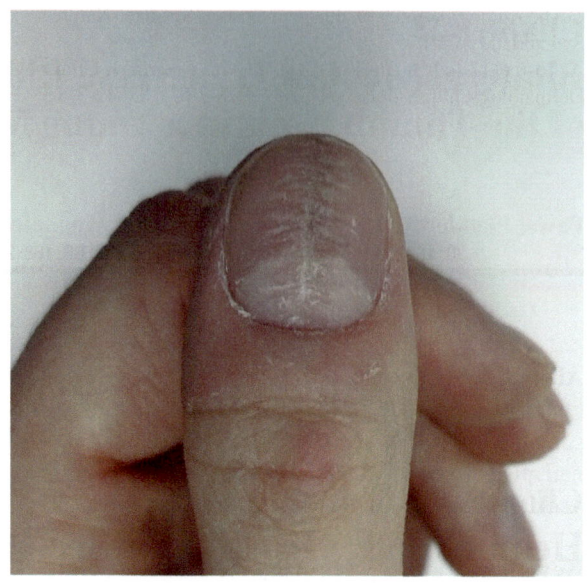

Dermatoscopic examination revealed irregular transverse indentations in the dorsal aspect of the nail plate, forming a median groove (Fig. 23.2).

Based on the Case Description and the Photographs, What Is Your Diagnosis?

1. Pterygium in the course of lichen planus
2. Bilateral trauma-induced nail dystrophy
3. Onychomatricoma
4. Nail psoriasis

Diagnosis

Bilateral trauma-induced nail dystrophy (median canaliform nail dystrophy of Heller/habit-tic deformity).

Fig. 23.2 Dermatoscopic presentation of the nail plate featuring central groove interconnected with radial transverse ridging affecting the lunula

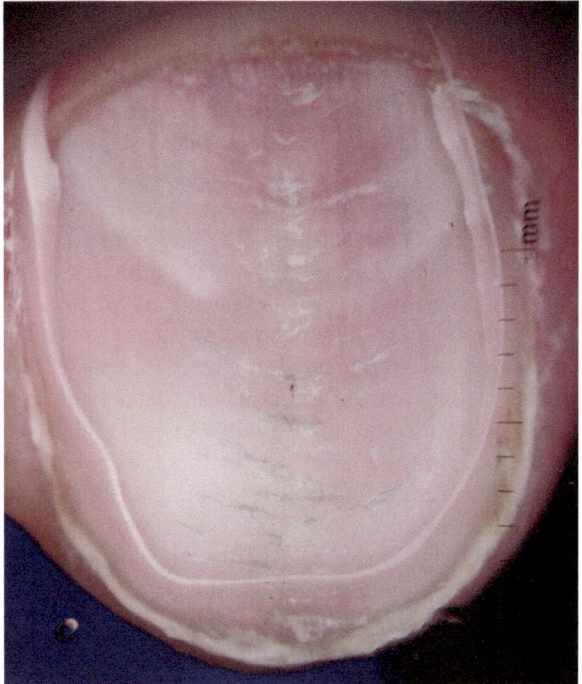

Discussion

When assessing bilateral morphological changes of the nail plates, it is crucial to collect a detailed history including possible systemic causes, occupation or the exact professional actions the patient is involved in, leisure, habits and tics, especially if the nail plate deformity is patterned (e.g. limited to particular fingernails or directly indicative of repetitive trauma). Onychoscopy is an auxiliary diagnostic method, increasing the diagnostic confidence and facilitating the differential diagnosis. Examination of the nail plate pigmentary disorders, conditions affecting the proximal nail fold or distal, free edge of the nail plate should be performed with polarized light and contact medium (optimally thick non-colored silicone gel) reducing the reflection and limiting the optical distortion caused by the nail plate curvature [1]. On the other hand, nail surface clues can be seen better with non-contact non-polarized dermatoscopy or non-contact ultraviolet-induced fluorescence dermatoscopy [1, 2].

Pterygium is a rare complication of lichen planus (LP) involving the nail unit. It is more common in advanced stages and estimated to develop in 4% of all LP patients, and 18–43% of those with isolated nail involvement [3]. LP is usually associated with nail matrix abnormalities (mainly longitudinal ridging and thinning of the nail plate), and less frequently nail bed abnormalities (onycholysis, hyperkeratosis, nail plate discoloration and crumbling) [3].

Onychomatricoma is a rare fibroepithelial tumor of the nail matrix, always affecting a single nail and occasionally painful. It is characterized by the gradually widening longitudinal chromonychia (usually yellow band, yet white or black can also occur) extending from under the proximal nail fold, nail plate thickening, proximal splinter hemorrhages, "honeycomb-like pattern" in axial assessment of the free distal edge, and overcurvature of the nail plate [4].

In psoriasis, transverse ridges and grooves within the nail plate (Beau's lines) form as a result of inflammation of the nail matrix and proximal nail folds, and are not specific for nail psoriasis but may develop in a number of dermatoses and systemic diseases [5]. They usually involve all fingernails or toenails, and extend laterally, occasionally resembling median canaliform nail dystrophy [1].

Median canaliform nail dystrophy of Heller (MCND), also known as onychodystrophia mediana canaliformis, nevus striatus unguis or solenonychia, is an uncommon nail disorder, presenting with transverse ridges that radiate from a paramedian groove or split [6]. Fissures or small cracks extend laterally from the central canal or split towards the nail edge resembling a Christmas tree or an inverted fir tree [6, 7]. Additionally, the lesion may be accompanied by the proximal nail fold erythema and thickening, as well as an enlarged lunula [8]. Histological characteristics of MCND include parakeratosis and inter- and intracellular melanin deposition in nail bed keratinocytes [6]. In the majority of cases, patients present with symmetrical involvement, and even though MCND usually affects the thumbnails, other fingernails or toenails may also be affected [6, 8]. No gender prevalence has been observed. A transient defective nail plate formation has been hypothesized to contribute to MCND, yet the exact etiopathogenesis remains unclear [6]. Despite the majority of MCND cases being apparently idiopathic, other plausible causes include repetitive trauma to the nail bed and/or nail plate, medications (e.g. oral retinoids, ritonavir, or others), focal infections and subungual tumors [6–10]. Trauma can be self-inflicted, such as nail biting, habit-tics, and scratching due to pruritic dermatoses [9]. While MCND is an acquired disorder, cases with familial clustering have also been reported [6].

The management of MCND is often challenging, with evidence limited to case reports. Treatment modalities include topical glucocorticosteroids (alone or combined with urea), flurandrenolide tape, intralesional triamcinolone acetonide injections, 0.1% tacrolimus ointment and 0.05% tazarotene ointment [6, 8, 9]. In secondary MCND, management of primary underlying disease is essential, e.g. dupilumab or Janus kinase inhibitors for atopic dermatitis. Some researchers noted the good response to multivitamins containing vitamin B2, B6, B7, C, E or laser treatment with 1064-nm Nd:YAG [8]. Cessation of culprit medication (isotretinoin, alitretinoin or ritonavir) accelerates the healing [9]. Short nail length and buffing the surface of the nail or covering the nail plate with a nail wrap/tape may provide a physical shield preventing further trauma. Furthermore, explaining the role of self-inflicted trauma in the development of MCND to the patient can increase self-awareness and better control [10]. Patients with habit-tics should be referred to a psychiatrist for counseling or antipsychotic treatment [9]. Cognitive behavioral therapy or habit reversal therapy should be also considered as non-pharmacologic interventions [10].

Key Points

- MCND is an uncommon nail disorder with paramedian ridge or split, and canal formation, that typically develops on both thumbnails. Most cases are deemed idiopathic, while nail bed and/or nail plate trauma, medications, nail infections and subungual tumors are further possible causes.
- To diagnose MCND, in addition to clinical examination and detailed history collection, onychoscopy can be utilized.
- Treatment options are not well established, but topical medications (corticosteroids, calcineurin inhibitors, urea and tazarotene), intralesional steroid injections, a few systemic agents (e.g. dupilumab, Janus kinase inhibitors and multivitamins), Nd:YAG laser, certain general measures (such as avoidance of further trauma with the application of a nail wrap/tape), and psychiatric counseling were reported to be effective in some instances.

References

1. Lallas A, Errichetti E, Ioannides D, editors. Dermoscopy in general dermatology. 1st ed. CRC Press; 2018. https://doi.org/10.1201/9781315201733.
2. Pietkiewicz P, Navarrete-Dechent C, Togawa Y, et al. Applications of ultraviolet and sub-ultraviolet dermatoscopy in neoplastic and non-neoplastic dermatoses: a systematic review. Dermatol Ther (Heidelb). 2024; https://doi.org/10.1007/s13555-024-01104-4. Published online February 15, 2024.
3. Żychowska M, Żychowska M. Nail changes in lichen planus: a single-center study. J Cutan Med Surg. 2021;25(3):281–5. https://doi.org/10.1177/1203475420982554.
4. Jaeger TNG, Canella C, Leverone AP, Nakamura RC. Onychomatricoma with onychomycosis: a case report and review of the literature. Skin Appendage Disord. 2021;7(5):422–6. https://doi.org/10.1159/000516662.
5. Pietkiewicz P, Bowszyc-Dmochowska M, Gornowicz-Porowska J, Dmochowski M. Involvement of nail apparatus in pemphigus vulgaris in ethnic poles is infrequent. Front Med (Lausanne). 2018;5:227. https://doi.org/10.3389/fmed.2018.00227.
6. Kota R, Pilani A, Nair PA. Median nail dystrophy involving the thumb nail. Indian J Dermatol. 2016;61(1):120. https://doi.org/10.4103/0019-5154.174092.
7. Madke B, Gadkari R, Nayak C. Median canaliform dystrophy of Heller. Indian Dermatol Online J. 2012;3(3):224–5. https://doi.org/10.4103/2229-5178.101832.
8. Quan EY, Johnson NM. Successful treatment of median canaliform nail dystrophy with topical tazarotene foam. JAAD Case Rep. 2022;29:70–1. https://doi.org/10.1016/j.jdcr.2022.08.051.

9. Wilson A, Tariq Khan M, Murrell DF. Median canaliform nail dystrophy in a 2-year-old boy: case report and review of the literature. Pediatr Dermatol. 2023;40(3):511–8. https://doi.org/10.1111/pde.15181.

10. Cohen PR. Nail-associated body-focused repetitive behaviors: habit-tic nail deformity, onychophagia, and onychotillomania. Cureus. 2022;14(3):e22818. https://doi.org/10.7759/cureus.22818.

Chapter 24
Monodactylic Longitudinal Melanonychia with a Hutchinson Sign in a Pentagenarian Woman

Paweł Pietkiewicz (ID) **and Adarsha Adhikari** (ID)

Abstract A pentagernarian woman presented with an isolated melanonychia of the third digit of the left hand. A 4 mm wide, brown band with irregularly-distributed, well-defined longitudinal parallel lines was visualized with onychoscopy. Gray-brownish structureless area extended from the cuticle to the proximal nail fold.

Keywords Melanonychia · Hutchinson sign · Congenital melanocytic nevus · Dermatoscopy · Onychoscopy

Clinical Case

A pentagenarian woman visited dermatology outpatients for a routine skin check-up. She had a Fitzpatrick skin type III and her personal medical history was noncontributory. During the examination, an isolated melanonychia of the third digit of her left hand was noted (Fig. 24.1). A dermatoscopic examination (Fig. 24.2) revealed a 4 mm wide, brown band with irregularly-distributed, well-defined longitudinal parallel lines extending from the proximal nail fold to the distal edge of the nail plate. Both the proximal nail fold and the cuticle exhibited hyperpigmentation in a form of gray-brownish structureless area. The distal edge of the nail and the surface of the nail plate were intact. There was no evidence of subungual hyperkeratosis (not shown). The patient noted no previous trauma and reported that the lesion had been present for as long as she could remember.

P. Pietkiewicz (✉)
Centrum Medyczne Zwierzyniecka, Poznań, Poland

A. Adhikari
Medical Private Practice, Pokhara, Nepal

Fig. 24.1 Clinical presentation of a single nail longitudinal melanonychia of a third digit in a pentagenarian woman

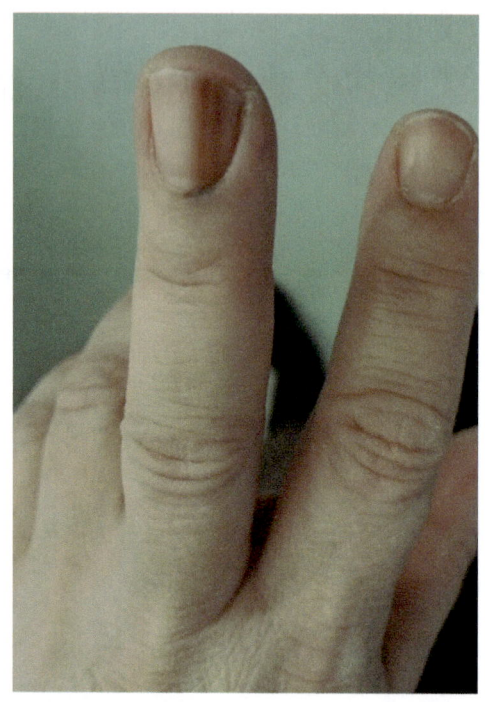

Fig. 24.2 Onychoscopic presentation of melanonychia

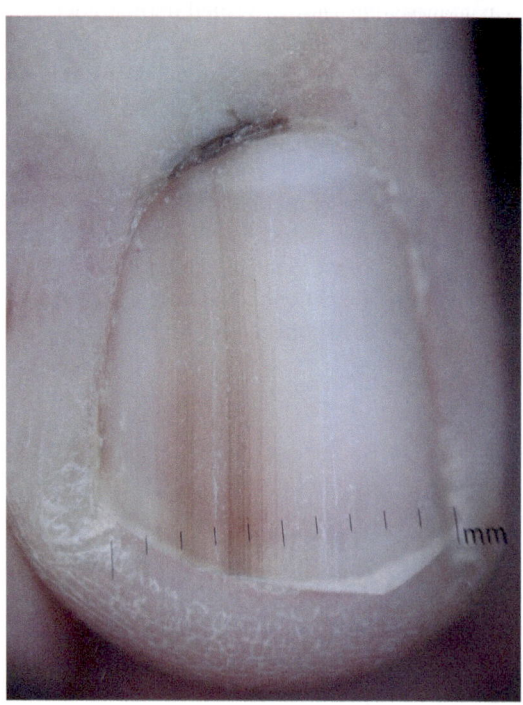

Based on the Case Description and the Photographs, What Is Your Diagnosis?

1. Subungual acral lentiginous melanoma
2. Congenital melanocytic nevus of the nail matrix
3. Pigmented intraepithelial carcinoma
4. Trauma-induced melanosis

Diagnosis

Congenital melanocytic nevus of the nail matrix

Discussion

Melanonychia refers to the pigmentation (black, brown, or gray) of the nail plate, often appearing as a longitudinal band [1]. It can develop due to benign and malignant conditions, including melanocyte activation and proliferation, infections, and trauma. It is important to consider subungual melanoma in every case of melanonychia.

A diagnostic biopsy for melanonychia can result in considerable trauma, painful healing, and potential deformation of the nail plate. Additionally, performing an excision too early, before the lesion meets the histological criteria for melanoma, might undermine the accuracy of the diagnosis. This is particularly relevant as lentiginous melanoma typically progresses very slowly. [2] Thus, an intelligent assessment of the dermatoscopic clues for melanoma is recommended, with a wait-and-see approach for non-obvious cases.

When assessing melanonychia, several variables need to be considered: the location of the lesion, the number of affected digits, the width and colour of the bands, the overall harmony of the lesion, the character of delineation, clues to growth, Hutchinson sign, any destruction of the nail plate, the presence of hemorrhages and the patient's history.

Subungual melanoma, accounting for about 0.7–3.5% of all melanoma cases, is relatively rare. However, its prevalence increases to 10–25% among Asians and Latinos and can reach up to 75% in individuals of African descent. [3] This type of melanoma most commonly affects the thumb or great toe nails (75–90% of cases), with the index finger being less commonly involved [3]. Thus, the occurrence of melanonychia at other sites generally argues against this diagnosis. Subungual melanoma is always isolated, whereas multiple affected nails are usually associated with ethnic pigmentation (darker skin types), drugs, hormonal stimulation, inflammatory diseases, trauma or syndromic conditions [3]. Nonetheless, monodactylic longitudinal melanonychia might also be associated with other conditions such as traumatic melanosis, nevus, lentigo, fungal infections, pigmented keratinocytic proliferations (like squamous cell carcinoma or onychomatricoma), or even the very rare subungual seborrheic keratosis. [2, 4, 5],

Single-colored, poorly defined gray bands in the nails are typically the result of lentigo, post-traumatic activation, ethnic factors, medication use, or certain syndromes. In contrast, when the pigmentation is brown, the primary considerations should be nevus or melanoma [2]. Mixed, multicoloured pigmentation is also more indicative for melanoma.

The general harmony related to width of bands and gaps between them, parallelism, uniformity of colour and delineation, tends to indicate a nevus. [1] In contrast, melanoma, as it grows and regresses, often shows signs of its dynamic nature. These signs include multicolored bands that are irregular in width and spacing, discontinuous, unevenly delineated, and sometimes arranged in a triangular shape pointing towards the distal edge of the nail plate, or associated with crumbling of the nail plate. The presence of longitudinal melanonychia, coupled with the simultaneous destruction of the nail apparatus, hemorrhages, and the Hutchinson sign, are key indicators of advanced subungual melanoma [6].

It's important to remember that the Hutchinson sign, often associated with melanoma, is not exclusively specific to this condition. It can also appear in cases of congenital or congenital-type nail matrix nevi, [7] as observed in this particular case. Therefore, the patient's history regarding the onset and development of the condition can be crucial in making an accurate diagnosis.

In the case of this patient, there was a monodactylic longitudinal brown melanonychia. Despite evident irregularity in colour and spacing, and co-existence with Hutchinson sign, early onset pointed to the diagnosis of congenital melanocytic nevus of the nail matrix. This diagnosis was further supported by the lack of any evolution in the condition over a long-term follow-up.

Key Points

- Dermatoscopy, while being a gold standard for assessing nail pigmentation, has limitations: congenital melanocytic nevi of the nail matrix can clinically and dermatoscopically mimic subungual melanomas.
- A comprehensive assessment of melanonychia involves several key variables: the lesion's location, the number of affected fingers, the width and color of the bands, general harmony of the lesion, the character of its delineation, clues to growth, the presence of Hutchinson's sign, nail plate destruction, hemorrhages, and last but not least, the patient's medical history.
- An onset during childhood and no evolution in adulthood in the course of long-term follow up typically confirm the benign nature of the pigmentation.

References

1. Starace M, Alessandrini A, Brandi N, Piraccini BM. Use of nail dermoscopy in the management of melanonychia: review. Dermatol Pract Concept. 2019;9(1):38–43. https://doi.org/10.5826/dpc.0901a10.
2. Lallas A, Korecka K, Apalla Z, et al. Seven plus one steps to assess pigmented nail bands (Melanonychia Striata Longitudinalis). Dermatol Pract Concept. 2023;13(4):e2023204. https://doi.org/10.5826/dpc.1304a204.
3. Mole RJ, MacKenzie DN. Subungual melanoma. In: StatPearls. StatPearls Publishing; 2023. Accessed 11 Jan 2024. http://www.ncbi.nlm.nih.gov/books/NBK482480/.
4. Jung SC, Lee TM, Kim M, Jo G, Mun JH. Pigmented onychomatricoma showing a longitudinal melanonychia: a case report and brief review of literature. Ann Dermatol. 2018;30(5):637–9. https://doi.org/10.5021/ad.2018.30.5.637.
5. Kameda E, Togawa Y, Maru Y, Matsue H. Ungual seborrheic keratosis with longitudinal melanonychia: a case report. J Dermatol. 2022;49(8):775–8. https://doi.org/10.1111/1346-8138.16392.
6. Wollina U, Tempel S, Hansel G. Subungual melanoma: a single center series from Dresden. Dermatol Ther. 2019;32(5):e13032. https://doi.org/10.1111/dth.13032.
7. Pham F, Boespflug A, Duru G, et al. Dermatoscopic and clinical features of congenital or congenital-type nail matrix nevi: a multicenter prospective cohort study by the International Dermoscopy Society. J Am Acad Dermatol. 2022;87(3):551–8. https://doi.org/10.1016/j.jaad.2022.01.028.

Chapter 25
Monodactylic Longitudinal Xanthonychia in a Middle-Aged Woman

Paweł Pietkiewicz ⓘ **and Ewelina Mazur** ⓘ

Abstract A yellowish-whitish longitudinal band developed on a third finger of the left hand of a middle-aged woman many months before the visit. The dermatoscopic examination of a thickened and crumbling nail plate revealed well-defined, longitudinal, parallel multicolored (yellow, white and red) bands extending from under the proximal nail fold to the distal edge. Partially translucent nail surface allowed visualization of elongated linear looped vessels parallel to the white bands.

Keywords Xanthonychia · Onychomatricoma · Nail tumor · Dermatoscopy · Onychoscopy

Clinical Case

A middle-aged woman (Fitzpatrick II) sought medical advice due to the slowly growing yellowish-whitish longitudinal band on a third finger of her left hand (Fig. 25.1). The lesion developed many months before the visit, and was slowly widening. No pain was reported by the patient, yet she was worried about the thickening and crumbling of the affected nail plate. There was no family history of skin cancer and her medical history was non-contributory. Dermatoscopic examination revealed well-defined, longitudinal, parallel multicolored (yellow, white and red)

P. Pietkiewicz (✉)
Centrum Medyczne Zwierzyniecka, Poznań, Poland

E. Mazur
Department of Dermatology, Institute of Medical Sciences, Medical College of Rzeszow University, Rzeszow, Poland

Doctoral School, University of Rzeszow, Rzeszow, Poland
e-mail: ewelinam@dokt.ur.edu.pl

© The Author(s), under exclusive license to Springer Nature Switzerland AG 2025
A. Tosti et al. (eds.), *Clinical Cases in Nail Disorders*, Clinical Cases in Dermatology, https://doi.org/10.1007/978-3-031-88642-3_25

145

Fig. 25.1 Monodactylic, asymptomatic yellowish-whitish discoloration present on the left third finger of a middle-aged woman

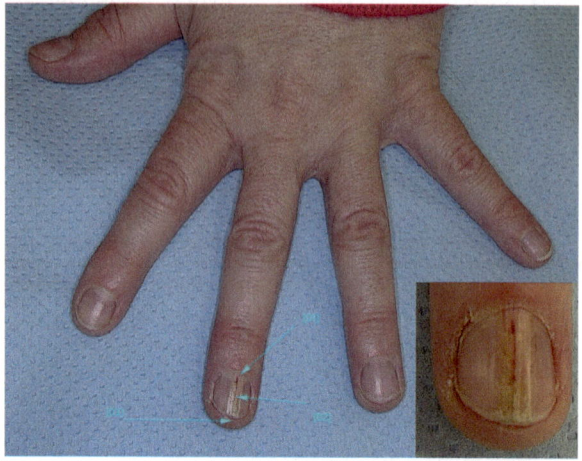

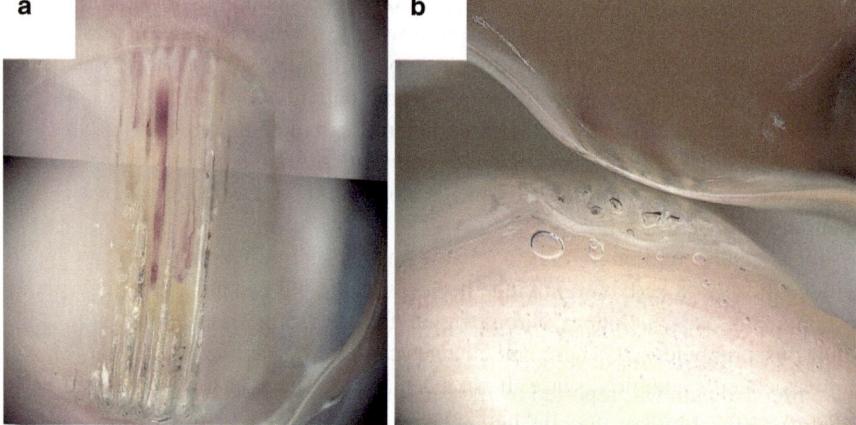

Fig. 25.2 Onychoscopy of a longitudinal striate xantho−/leukonychia of the left third finger of a middle aged woman. (**a**) Yellowish-whitish longitudinal band of uniform width, extending from the nail matrix, and proximally displaying elongated linear looped vessels and hemorrhages. Note the parallel and well-defined lateral edges, as well as the crumbling of the distal free edge of the nail plate. (**b**) Axial onychoscopy of the free distal nail edge exhibits thickening of the nail plate with a distinctive "honeycomb-like pattern" and no subungual hyperkeratosis

bands extending from under the proximal nail fold to the distal edge (Fig. 25.2a). Partially translucent nail surface allowed visualization of elongated linear looped vessels parallel to the white bands. The proximal surface of the nail was not affected, whereas the distal surface displayed linear pitting and crumbling of the free edge. Axial onychoscopy demonstrated thickening of the free edge, interrupted with roundish foramina (Fig. 25.2b).

Based on the Case Description and the Photographs, What Is Your Diagnosis?

1. Subungual exostosis
2. Onychomatricoma
3. Onychopapilloma
4. Squamous cell carcinoma

Diagnosis

Onychomatricoma

Discussion

Onychomatricoma (OM) represents a rare, predominantly asymptomatic, and slow-growing fibroepithelial tumor of the nail matrix. It usually affects adults and has no ethnic or sex predilection. The incidence in fingernails is thrice as common as in toenails. OM grows longitudinally toward the distal nail plate edge with multiple digitate fibroepithelial projections. Clinically, it is usually characterized by 4 major features: longitudinal xanthonychia, proximal splinter hemorrhages, thickening of the nail plate, and transverse overcurvature of the nail plate [1].

Differential diagnosis includes subungual squamous cell carcinoma (suSCC), fibrokeratoma, onychomycosis, osteochondroma, and subungual wart. Since suSCC presents mostly as distal onycholysis, subungual hyperkeratosis, and nail color changes (leukonychia, erythronychia, xanthonychia), in some cases making a straightforward clinical diagnosis between suSCC and OM can be challenging and may require onychoscopy. OM is also one of the three nail tumors (along with rare onychocytic matricoma and onychocytic carcinoma) presenting as pachyonychia striata [2]. It usually features thickened nail plate and well-defined parallel lateral edges, whereas suSCC prevalently features subungual hyperkeratosis and nonparallel lateral lesion edges (referred to as polycyclic or fuzzy) [3, 4].

Onychopapilloma is a benign neoplasm that can originate either from the distal nail matrix or the proximal nail bed. It is characterized by longitudinal erythronychia with splinter hemorrhages, notch in lunula, V-shaped fissuring of a distal nail plate and a subungual filiform hyperkeratosis. Since early onychopapilloma may mimic OM, dermoscopy of the free edge of the distal nail plate (esp. the presence of honeycomb-like cavitations in OM) is of great value [5, 6].

Of note, as pigmented OM presents as longitudinal melanonychia, it may simulate perfectly subungual melanoma, pigmented subungual intraepithelial carcinoma, or fungal melanonychia [7].

Histologic criteria of OM include: (1) presence of fibroepithelial tumor composed of 2 portions: proximal with pedunculated base, and distal with multiple digitate projections; (2) a 2-layered stroma with superficial being more cellular, and deeper featuring thicker collagen bundles; (3) a thick keratogenous V-shaped zone present at the level of epithelial ridges, both proximally and distally, forming a thickened nail plate [8]. A nail clipping technique is a minimally invasive method used to confirm the diagnosis. The clippings usually reveal lacunae filled with serous fluid, responsible for the "honeycomb-like pattern" or a "woodworm-like cavitation" observed in the nail free edge onychoscopy [2, 6]. Periodic acid–Schiff stain can be used to rule out onychomycosis. In instances where onychomatricoma specimens are sent to the pathologist without the nail plate precise diagnosis can be challenging and may require additional immunohistochemical studies (e.g. CD10, CD13, CD34, AE13, and LEF-1) for reliable differentiation of OM from various superficial fibrous tumors [1, 8, 9]. Imaging studies with ultrasonography, radiography, magnetic resonance imaging, reflectance confocal microscopy, and optical coherence tomography can aid the diagnosis [10].

Key Points

- Onychomatricoma is a rare tumor of the nail matrix, usually affecting the fingernails and presenting with longitudinal xanthonychia, proximal splinter hemorrhages, thickening of the nail plate, and transverse overcurvature of the nail plate.
- Differential diagnosis of onychomatricoma includes squamous cell carcinoma, onychopapilloma, fibrokeratoma, onychomycosis, osteochondroma, and subungual wart.
- Onychoscopy is an auxiliary diagnostic technique facilitating the diagnosis of onychomatricoma, as the tumor usually displays well-defined border with parallel lateral edges, and distal free edge presenting with "honeycomb-like pattern" ungual hyperkeratosis.

References

1. Jaeger TNG, Canella C, Leverone AP, Nakamura RC. Onychomatricoma with onychomycosis: a case report and review of the literature. Skin Appendage Disord. 2021;7(5):422–6. https://doi.org/10.1159/000516662.
2. Perrin C, Cannata GE, Langbein L, et al. Acquired localized longitudinal pachyonychia and onychomatrical tumors: a comparative study to onychomatricomas (5 cases) and onychocytic matricomas (4 cases). Am J Dermatopathol. 2016;38(9):664–71. https://doi.org/10.1097/DAD.0000000000000511.
3. Lesort C, Debarbieux S, Duru G, Dalle S, Poulhalon N, Thomas L. Dermoscopic features of onychomatricoma: a study of 34 cases. Dermatology. 2015;231(2):177–83. https://doi.org/10.1159/000431315.

4. Teysseire S, Dalle S, Duru G, et al. Dermoscopic features of subungual squamous cell carcinoma: a study of 44 cases. Dermatology. 2017;233(2–3):184–91. https://doi.org/10.1159/000479059.
5. Tosti A, Schneider SL, Ramirez-Quizon MN, Zaiac M, Miteva M. Clinical, dermoscopic, and pathologic features of onychopapilloma: a review of 47 cases. J Am Acad Dermatol. 2016;74(3):521–6. https://doi.org/10.1016/j.jaad.2015.08.053.
6. Oak ASW, Elewski BE, Pavlidakey PG, Mayo TT. Honeycomb-like cavities in a single fingernail plate. JAAD Case Rep. 2020;6(2):89–91. https://doi.org/10.1016/j.jdcr.2019.10.019.
7. Isales MC, Haugh AM, Bubley J, et al. Pigmented onychomatricoma: a rare mimic of subungual melanoma. Clin Exp Dermatol. 2018;43(5):623–6. https://doi.org/10.1111/ced.13418.
8. Perrin C, Baran R, Pisani A, Ortonne JP, Michiels JF. The onychomatricoma: additional histologic criteria and immunohistochemical study. Am J Dermatopathol. 2002;24(3):199–203. https://doi.org/10.1097/00000372-200206000-00002.
9. Perrin C, Pedeutour F, Coutts M, Ambrosetti D, Dadone-Montaudié B. Onychomatricoma: a clinicopathological, immunohistochemical, and molecular study of 10 cases highlighting recurrent RB1 deletion and the potential diagnostic value of LEF-1. Histopathology. 2023;82(5):767–78. https://doi.org/10.1111/his.14864.
10. Cinotti E, Veronesi G, Labeille B, et al. Imaging technique for the diagnosis of onychomatricoma. J Eur Acad Dermatol Venereol. 2018;32(11):1874–8. https://doi.org/10.1111/jdv.15108.

Chapter 26
Twenty-Nail Transverse Leuko- and Melanonychia Striata in Elderly Man

Paweł Pietkiewicz ⓘ **and Adarsha Adhikari** ⓘ

Abstract An octogenarian man, a locksmith by occupation, presented to the dermatology outpatients due to 1 month history of twenty–nail changes. The surface of the nails was uneven, characterized by regular transverse ridges and alternating brown and white transverse bands. The remembered that the nail changes were preceded by the severe itch by 2 months. Dermatoscopic assessment revealed confirmed transverse melanonychia and leukonychia striata that did not change under pressure.

Keywords Twenty nail dystrophy · Chemotherapy · Anti-cancer drugs · Melanonychia · Leukonychia striata

Clinical Case

An octogenarian man, a locksmith by occupation, presented to the dermatology outpatients due to twenty–nail changes (Figs. 26.1 and 26.2). The surface of the nails was uneven, characterized by regular transverse ridges (known as Beau's lines) and alternating brown and white transverse bands. He reported that these nail changes first appeared approximately 1 month prior to his consultation. Moreover, he described experiencing severe itch that began 2 months ago. The patient had a medical history of hypertension, hypercholesterolaemia and prostate hypertrophy, and was participating in a clinical trial for the treatment of acute myeloid leukemia. While he could not remember all the medications he was taking, he did recall using

P. Pietkiewicz (✉)
Centrum Medyczne Zwierzyniecka, Poznań, Poland

A. Adhikari
Medical Private Practice, Pokhara, Nepal

© The Author(s), under exclusive license to Springer Nature Switzerland AG 2025
A. Tosti et al. (eds.), *Clinical Cases in Nail Disorders*, Clinical Cases in Dermatology, https://doi.org/10.1007/978-3-031-88642-3_26

151

eplerenone. Documentation from the clinical trial (NCT03151408) indicated that that he was receiving azacitidine (administered at a dose of 75 mg/m² daily for 7 days during a cycle of 28 days) and either a placebo or pracinostat (administered at a dose of 60 mg daily, 3 days a week, for 3 weeks in a row during a cycle of 28 days) for the past 6 months.

Dermatoscopic assessment revealed confirmed transverse melanonychia and leukonychia striata that did not change under pressure (Fig. 26.3). The cuticle remained spared from pigmentation and there was no evidence of subungual hyperkeratosis.

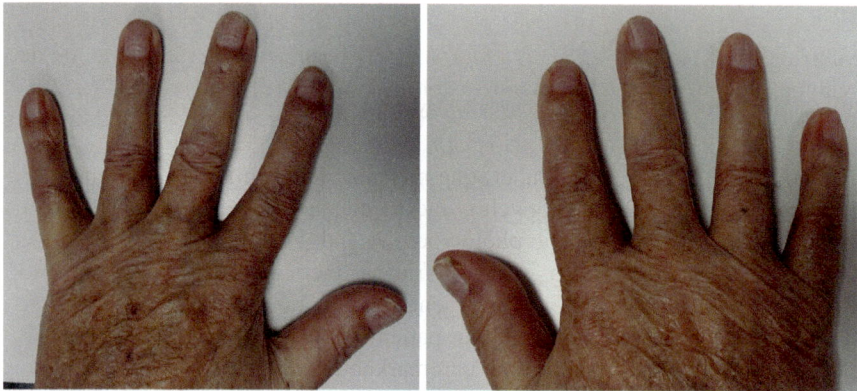

Fig. 26.1 Clinical presentation of pigmentation disorder of twenty nails in an octogenarian man

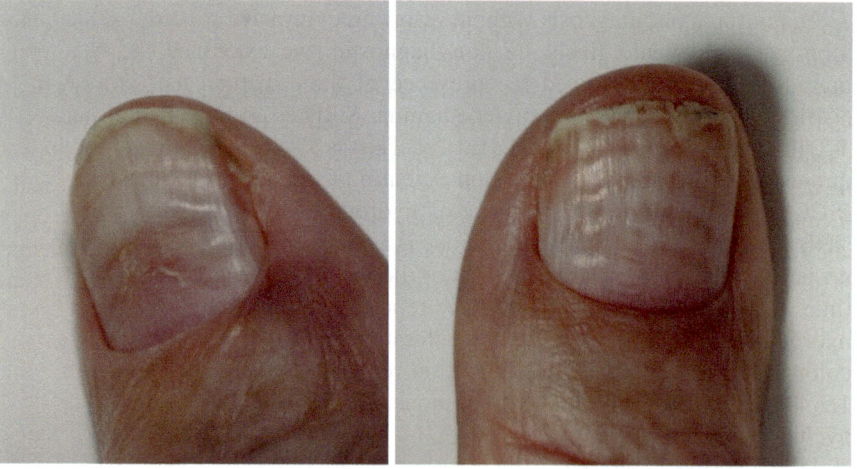

Fig. 26.2 Regular transverse alternate white and brown bands of the nail bed and transverse ridging of the dorsal aspect of the nail plate

Fig. 26.3 Onychoscopic
presentation of transverse
leuko- and melanonychia
striata and Beau's lines

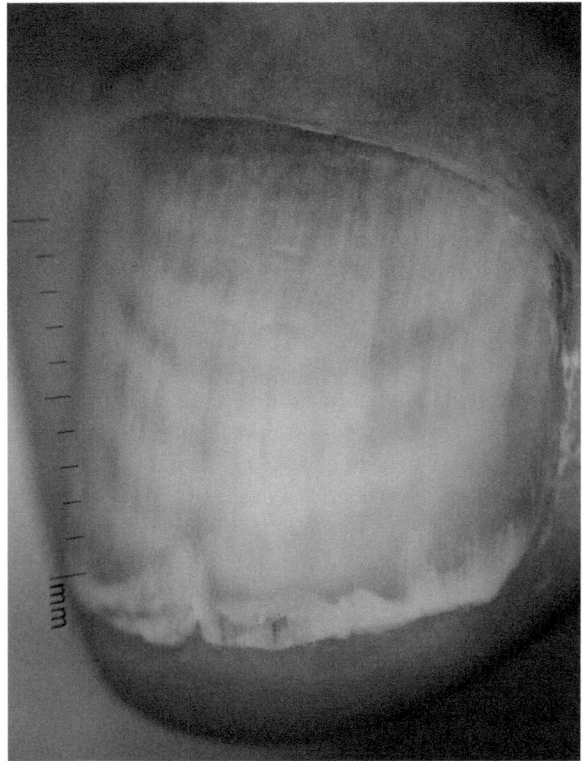

Based on the Case Description and the Photographs, What Is Your Diagnosis?

1. Twenty-nail dystrophy
2. Chemotherapy-induced nail changes
3. Heavy metal poisoning
4. Trauma-induced melanosis

Diagnosis

Chemotherapy-induced nail changes

Discussion

Twenty-nail dystrophy is a rare condition with unknown etiology, usually developing in childhood. It features longitudinal ridging, trachyonychia (roughness) and occasionally pitting. Nonetheless, it can be associated with a range of conditions, including chemotherapy [1]. In the described patient, there was neither loss of nail plate mirror, nor longitudinal ridging.

Beau's lines are transverse, linear depressions of the dorsal nail plate caused by the transient inhibition of mitotic activity of keratinocytes of the proximal nail matrix [2]. Along with a transverse leukonychia that does not fade with compression (Mees' lines, true leukonychia), but is localized within the nail plate, Beau's lines can develop with heavy metal poisoning (e.g. with arsenium, cadmium, thalium, selenium, mercury or others) or develop due to any antimitotic drug [2, 3]. In this case, the transverse leukonychia seemed unrelated to the nail matrix, but rather associated with disrupted vascularity of the nail bed (Muehrcke's lines, apparent leukonychia) [3].

Trauma-induced melanosis originates from matrix melanocyte activation due to acute or chronic physical triggers (sports, occupational trauma, dancing, ill-fitted shoes) and is usually limited to a single of a few nails, exhibiting longitudinal—not transverse, grayish bands. Multiple nails affected may indicate ethnic, drug-induced or syndromic background [4].

Cutaneous adverse effects can develop due to chemotherapeutic agents, whereas nail toxicity is the most frequent one, occurring in the course of both newer and classical drug [5]. Azacitidine is a cytidine analogue used for the treatment of acute myeloid leukemia (AML) and myelodysplastic syndromes (MDSs) in older adults, with two-faceted antineoplastic activity. The drug directly inhibits DNA methyltransferases which leads to p53-independent apoptosis; and binds RNA, ultimately leading to the inhibition of the production of proteins in a tumor cell [6]. Pracinostat is a dialkyl benzimidazole, a histone deacetylase competitive inhibitor [7]. Combined therapy of azacitidine and pracinostat is an effective and well-tolerated synergistic anticancer regimen used as first line treatment in older AML patients, who are not candidates for intense therapy [6, 7]. Chemotherapy-induced nail dystrophy and transverse pigmented bands are common (Table 26.1). Of note, these pigmentary changes usually manifest after several weeks to months of treatment, likely do not correspond to true Muehrcke's nails (typically related to hypoalbuminemia), and have a tendency to resolve with treatment cessation [3, 8].

Table 26.1 Chemotherapeutic agents commonly associated with nail abnormalities

Mees' lines (true leukonychia)	Cyclophosphamide, doxorubicin, vincristine, docetaxel, paclitaxel, combination of cytarabine/ daunorubicin [5]
Muehrcke's lines (apparent leukonychia)	Combination of cyclophosphamide/ doxorubicin/5-fluorouracil, combination of vincristine/doxorubicin/dexamethasone, cisplatin, oxaliplatin [5]
Beau's lines	Cyclophosphamide, vincristine, bleomycin, tegafur, combination of cyclophosphamide/ adriamycin/vincristine [5], paclitaxel, docetaxel [7], dapsone and octreotide [2]
Longitudinal melanonychia	Cyclophosphamide, vincristine, bleomycin, tegafur, adriamycin, vincristine, imatinib [5]
Diffuse melanonychia	Cyclophosphamide, vincristine, capecitabine, cisplatin, carboplatin, oxaliplatin, 5-fluorouracil, doxorubicin, daunorubicin, adriamycin, bleomycin, hydroxycarbamide (hydroxyurea), busulfan, docetaxel, paclitaxel, pemetrexed, etoposide, [5] imatinib [8]

Key Points

- Twenty-nail changes are related to systemic condition or drug. Regular transverse changes in color and/or surface of the dorsal aspect of the nail plate reflex the intervals in which culprit drug interferes with the growth of the nail matrix.
- Low albumin level is usually associated with apparent leukonychia (responsive to digital pressure, and unrelated to nail matrix) in non-oncological patients.
- Chemotherapy-associate alternate transverse pigmented bands of the nail bed (e.g. leukonychia or melanonychia) in oncological patients may develop weeks to months after the initiation of therapy and resolve upon its discontinuation.

References

1. Jacobsen AA, Tosti A. Trachyonychia and twenty-nail dystrophy: a comprehensive review and discussion of diagnostic accuracy. Skin Appendage Disord. 2016;2(1–2):7–13. https://doi.org/10.1159/000445544.
2. Wollina U, Abdel-Naser MB. Drug reactions affecting hair and nails. Clin Dermatol. 2020;38(6):693–701. https://doi.org/10.1016/j.clindermatol.2020.06.009.
3. Ramachandran V, Sapra A. Muehrcke lines of the fingernails. In: StatPearls. StatPearls Publishing; 2024. Accessed 26 Jan 2024. http://www.ncbi.nlm.nih.gov/books/NBK559136/.
4. Singal A, Bisherwal K. Melanonychia: etiology, diagnosis, and treatment. Indian Dermatol Online J. 2020;11(1):1–11. https://doi.org/10.4103/idoj.IDOJ_167_19.
5. Emvalomati A, Oflidou V, Papageorgiou C, et al. Narrative review of drug-associated nail toxicities in oncologic patients. Dermatol Pract Concept. 2023;13(1):e2023064. https://doi.org/10.5826/dpc.1301a64.
6. Montalban-Bravo G, Garcia-Manero G. Novel drugs for older patients with acute myeloid leukemia. Leukemia. 2015;29(4):760–9. https://doi.org/10.1038/leu.2014.244.
7. Huang TC, Chao TY. Mees lines and Beau lines after chemotherapy. CMAJ. 2010;182(3):E149. https://doi.org/10.1503/cmaj.090501.
8. Sanmartín O, Beato C, Suh-Oh HJ, et al. Clinical management of cutaneous adverse events in patients on chemotherapy: a national consensus statement by the Spanish academy of dermatology and venereology and the Spanish society of medical oncology. Actas Dermosifiliogr (Engl Ed). 2019;110(6):448–59. https://doi.org/10.1016/j.adengl.2019.05.003.

Chapter 27
Unraveling Neurological Disorders Through Dermatological Signs

Michela Starace ⓘ, **Stephano Cedirian** ⓘ, **Federico Quadrelli** ⓘ, **and Bianca Maria Piraccini** ⓘ

Abstract Carpal Tunnel Syndrome (CTS) is widely recognized for its neurological implications but less so for its dermatological manifestations. This case highlights an 89-year-old woman presenting with erosive, non-healing lesions and nail abnormalities in the fingers innervated by the median nerve. Clinical examination and diagnostic tests confirmed CTS with associated acroosteolysis and trophic changes in the skin and nails. The findings emphasize the importance of considering CTS in differential diagnoses of cutaneous and nail abnormalities, particularly when neurological symptoms coexist. Early recognition and management of these atypical manifestations are critical for comprehensive care.

Keywords Carpal tunnel syndrome · Nail abnormalities in CTS · Cutaneous abnormalities in CTS · Median nerve neuropathy · Dermatosis in neurological disorders

Clinical Case

An 89-year-old woman presented with an erosive non-healing lesion on the tip and the fingernail of the third digit of the left hand appeared 6 months before (Fig. 27.1). Clinical examination revealed a shortened distal phalanx with a short and thin nail as well as periungual crusts. Onychoscopy revealed a short nail plate, blurred brown

M. Starace · S. Cedirian (✉) · F. Quadrelli · B. M. Piraccini
Dermatology Unit, IRCCS Azienda Ospedaliero-Universitaria di Bologna, Bologna, Italy

Department of Medical and Surgical Sciences, Alma Mater Studiorum University of Bologna, Bologna, Italy
e-mail: michela.starace2@unibo.it; federico.quadrelli3@studio.unibo.it; biancamaria.piraccini@unibo.it

© The Author(s), under exclusive license to Springer Nature Switzerland AG 2025
A. Tosti et al. (eds.), *Clinical Cases in Nail Disorders*, Clinical Cases in Dermatology, https://doi.org/10.1007/978-3-031-88642-3_27

in color, with multiple splinter hemorrhages, mild subungual hyperkeratosis and periungual hematic crusts (Fig. 27.2). Careful examination allowed identification of another small subungual erosion on the second fingernail of the same hand (Fig. 27.3) and observation of the palmar skin revealed an additional skin erosion on the ventrolateral side of the second left digit (Fig. 27.4).

Additionally, the patient reported that the lesions were devoid of pain, but she complained of nocturnal paresthesias and hypoesthesia in the first three fingers of her left hand since the previous year. Thumb opposition and thenar atrophy (Fig. 27.5) were also noted, alongside positive Tinel's and Phalen's maneuvers.

A Doppler Ultrasound of the upper limbs demonstrated normal blood flow, while X-ray imaging revealed acroosteolysis of the distal phalanx of the of the third digit (Fig. 27.6). A neurologic consultation and electroneurography examination confirmed the presence of left median nerve neuropathy.

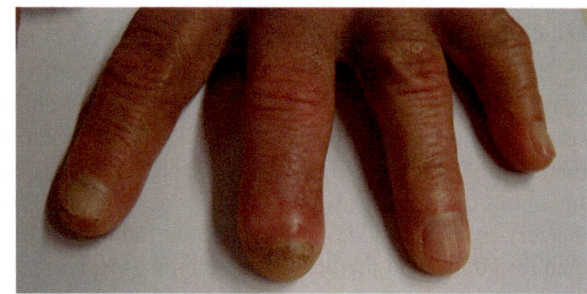

Fig. 27.1 Clinical image revealing erosive lesions of the tip of third digits, along with shortening of the distal phalanx

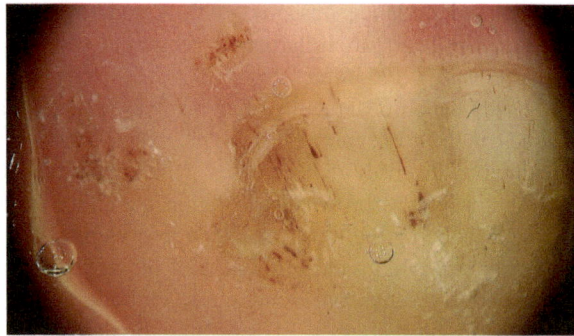

Fig. 27.2 Onychoscopy shows a short, thin, brownish nail plate with splinter hemorrhages and periungual blood crusts. A closer clinical examination showcasing the erosive, non-healing lesions on the ventrolateral aspect of the second left digit

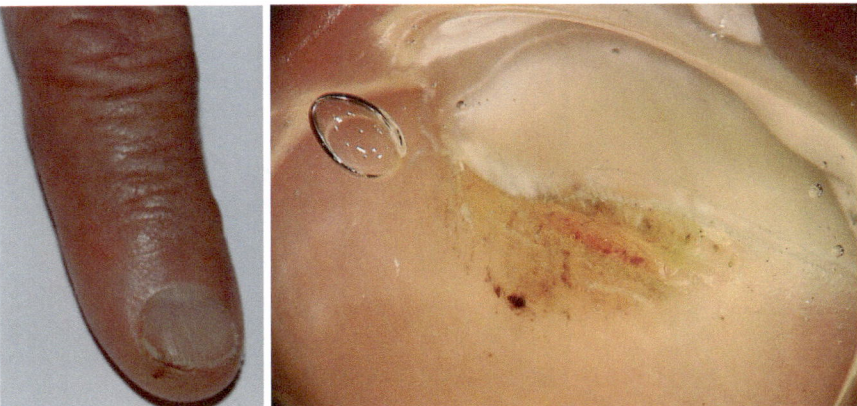

Fig. 27.3 The second fingernail shows a subungual erosion, better identified by onychoscopy

Fig. 27.4 Skin erosion of the ventral surface of the second finger. Co-presence of thenar atrophy noted on the left hand

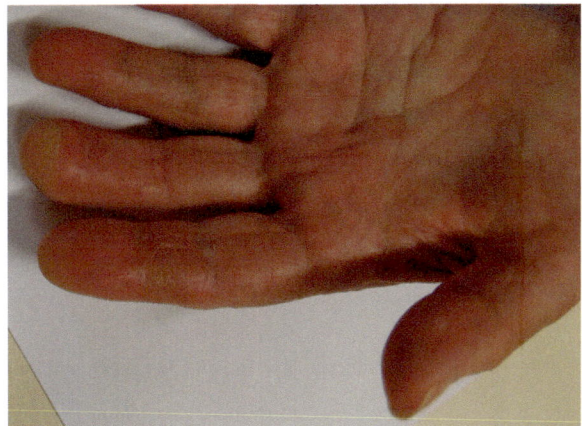

Fig. 27.5 Atrophy of the thenar muscle of the right hand

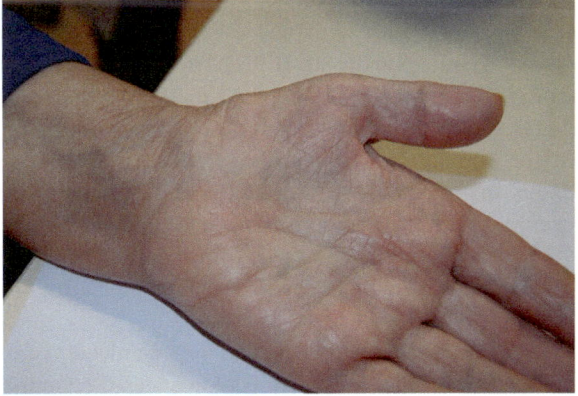

Fig. 27.6 Xray of the right hand showing massive acroosteolysis of the third finger

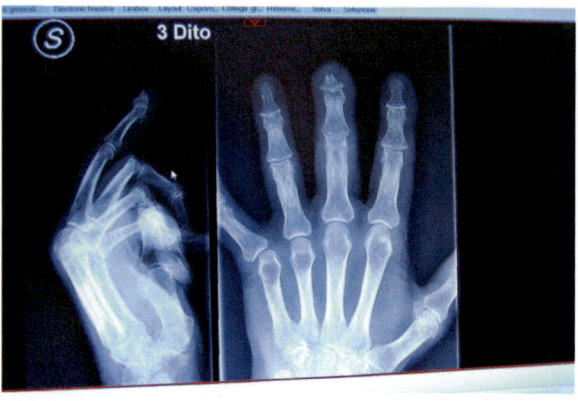

Based on the Case Description and the Photographs, What Is Your Diagnosis?

1. Winiwarter-Buerger Disease
2. Diabetic Neuropathy
3. Nail squamous cell carcinoma
4. Carpal Tunnel Syndrome

Diagnosis

Cutaneous and nail alterations due to carpal tunnel syndrome (CTS).

Discussion

Carpal Tunnel Syndrome (CTS) affects a significant portion of adults, ranging from 0.1% to 0.6% of the population [1]. This condition is characterized by the compression of the median nerve within the carpal tunnel, resulting in sensory, motor, and autonomic neural dysfunctions [2–4]. Literature exploring the cutaneous manifestations of CTS remains relatively limited; however, there is a growing focus and attention on this topic [1, 2]. The dermatological effects of CTS arise from vasomotor dysfunction and insufficient vascular supply to the median nerve due to mechanical pressure, leading to trophic changes in the skin and nails [5].

Dermatological manifestations include ulcers, xerosis, erosions, digital edema, and nail abnormalities [1, 6]. Nail changes predominantly affect the first, second, and third digits of the afflicted hand [1].

Nail changes seen in CTS are characterized by a wide spectrum of alterations: Beau's lines, melanonychia, leukonychia, onycholysis, koilonychia, and onychomadesis typically characterize mild forms [1, 6]. On the other hand, thickened, keratotic nails, alongside peri- and subungual ischemic lesions, paronychia, and acro-osteolysis characterize severe CTS forms [1].

The differential diagnosis should carefully consider other causes of peripheral nerve damage that may present with similar clinical characteristics to CTS [7–9]. Conditions such as diabetes or vascular disorders like Winiwarter-Buerger disease [7–9] should be taken into account. Buerger's syndrome, for instance, is distinguished by chronic paronychia, proximal leukonychia, onycholysis, and nail bed erosion, all of which can serve as early indicators of vascular involvement in the disease [9]. Recognizing these nail abnormalities is paramount for prompt diagnosis and intervention [9]. Another condition that may resemble nail involvement in CTS, albeit not directly associated with nerve damage, is nail unit squamous cell carcinoma (NU-SCC) [10]. NU-SCC may present as a digital painless ulcer with a diverse range of dermoscopic features, including vascular structures, such as milky-red areas, linear, coiled and arborizing vessels, along with whitish scaly areas, yellowish scales and dots [10].

Intriguingly, the specific type of nail abnormality in CTS does not suggest the diagnosis; rather, it is the distribution of these changes along the pathway of the median nerve, namely the involvement of the first 3 digits and fingernails, along with the history of paresthesia and nocturnal pain [1].

The management of dermatological conditions in CTS is linked to effectively managing CTS itself [1]. For mild cases, treatment options include the use of wrist splints and corticosteroid injections. Additionally, topical application of nitroglycerin patches can aid in addressing skin and nail necrotic lesions [1]. However, the most effective and definitive treatment for CTS involves surgical decompression of the median nerve [3, 4]. Surgical options include open carpal tunnel release and endoscopic carpal tunnel release: these procedures aim to alleviate pressure on the median nerve, thereby providing relief from CTS symptoms and potentially improving associated dermatological manifestations [3, 4].

In conclusion, CTS extends beyond its well-known neurological symptoms. Nail and skin alterations, arising from vasomotor dysfunction, temporary vasospasms, and inadequate vascularization, are significant components of CTS that demand attention. Dermatologists play a pivotal role in recognizing and managing these effects, thereby contributing to comprehensive care for individuals with CTS.

Key Points

1. **Dermatological Manifestations of CTS:** CTS, primarily recognized for its neurological symptoms, can also manifest dermatological alterations such as ulcers, xerosis, erosions, digital edema, and nail abnormalities. These changes stem from vasomotor dysfunction and inadequate vascular supply to the median nerve due to mechanical pressure within the carpal tunnel.

2. **Differential Diagnosis Consideration:** When evaluating dermatological alterations in the context of peripheral nerve damage, clinicians must differentiate CTS from other conditions such as diabetes, and vascular disorders like Winiwarter-Buerger disease. Additionally, certain mimicking conditions like NU-SCC should always be considered and ruled out. Understanding the distinct nail abnormalities associated with each condition aids in accurate diagnosis and timely intervention.

References

1. Egger A, Tosti A. Carpal tunnel syndrome and associated nail changes: review and examples from the author's practice. J Am Acad Dermatol. 2020;83(6):1724–9. https://doi.org/10.1016/j.jaad.2020.03.023.
2. Soares C, Teixeira V, Santos-Faria D. Digital ulcers and shortening of the second and third fingers as manifestations of carpal tunnel syndrome. Int J Dermatol. 2024;63(2):244–5. https://doi.org/10.1111/ijd.16893.
3. Petrover D, Richette P. Treatment of carpal tunnel syndrome: from ultrasonography to ultrasound guided carpal tunnel release. Joint Bone Spine. 2018;85(5):545–52. https://doi.org/10.1016/j.jbspin.2017.11.003.
4. Karamanos E, Jillian BQ, Person D. Endoscopic carpal tunnel release: indications, technique, and outcomes. Orthop Clin North Am. 2020;51(3):361–8. https://doi.org/10.1016/j.ocl.2020.02.001.
5. Reddeppa S, Bulusu K, Chand PR, Jacob PC, Kalappurakkal J, Tharakan J. The sympathetic skin response in carpal tunnel syndrome. Auton Neurosci. 2000;84(3):119–21. https://doi.org/10.1016/S1566-0702(00)00190-9.
6. Cho SB, Lee SH, Kim J. Koilonychia in carpal-tunnel syndrome. Clin Exp Dermatol. 2010;35(4):e145–6. https://doi.org/10.1111/j.1365-2230.2009.03720.x.
7. Greene RA, Scher RK. Nail changes associated with diabetes mellitus. J Am Acad Dermatol. 1987;16(5 Pt 1):1015–21. https://doi.org/10.1016/s0190-9622(87)70131-5.
8. Mazereeuw-Hautier J, Bonafé JL. Bilateral Beau's lines and pyogenic granulomas following Guillain-Barré syndrome. Dermatology. 2004;209(3):237–8. https://doi.org/10.1159/000079898.
9. Starace MVR, Alessandrini A, Tosti A, Piraccini BM. Nails involvement in winiwarter-buerger disease. Skin Appendage Disord. 2022;8(2):142–5. https://doi.org/10.1159/000518982.
10. Starace M, Alessandrini A, Dika E, Piraccini BM. Squamous cell carcinoma of the nail unit. Dermatol Pract Concept. 2018;8(3):238–44. https://doi.org/10.5826/dpc.0803a17. Published 2018 July 31.

Chapter 28
"A Red Subungual Mass"

Florence Dehavay, Marisa Mathieu, Charlotte Arnal, Marie Caucanas, Florine Moulart, and Bertrand Richert Baran

Abstract This clinical case discusses the various causes of nodule on the nail bed. It highlights that physicians should keep in mind a possible malignant cause and always biopsy the lesion.

Keywords Subungual pyogenic granuloma · Squamous cell carcinoma · Amelanotic melanoma

F. Dehavay · M. Mathieu · B. Richert Baran (✉)
Department of Dermatology, University Hospital Saint Pierre, Université Libre de Bruxelles, Brussels, Belgium
e-mail: Bertrand.richert@chu-brugmann.be

C. Arnal
Department of Dermatology, Université de Lorraine, Nancy, France

M. Caucanas
Clinique des Minimes, Toulouse, France

F. Moulart
Department of Dermatology, University Hospital Saint Pierre, Université Libre de Bruxelles, Brussels, Belgium

Department of Dermatology, Clinique Notre-Dame de Grâce, Gosselies, Belgium
e-mail: Florine.Moulart@ulb.be

Clinical Case

A 73-year-old male, with no significant history other than a long-standing smoking habit, consulted for a progressive, painless alteration of his right thumbnail that had been evolving for 5 years. A recent trauma had led to significant bleeding, prompting him to seek medical advice. Clinical examination revealed an enlargement of the distal phalanx of the right thumb, with extensive onycholysis of the lateral half of the nail plate, associated with a fleshy subungual lesion (Figs. 28.1 and 28.2). Clipping of the detached plate revealed an erythematous, bleeding, non-specific proliferating tumour. Dermatoscopy showed an atypical vascular pattern with no pigmentation.

Fig. 28.1 Nodular fleshy lesion of the bed after clipping of the detached plate

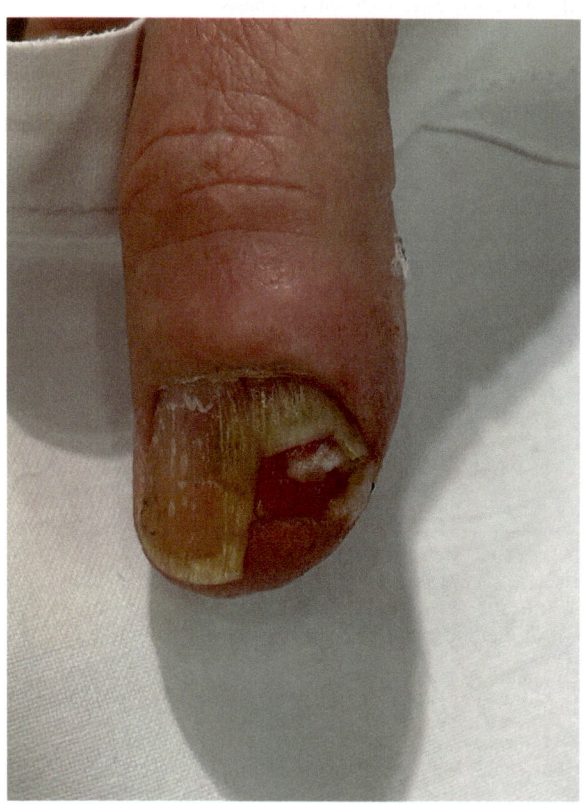

Fig. 28.2 Dermatoscopy
aspect of the lesion

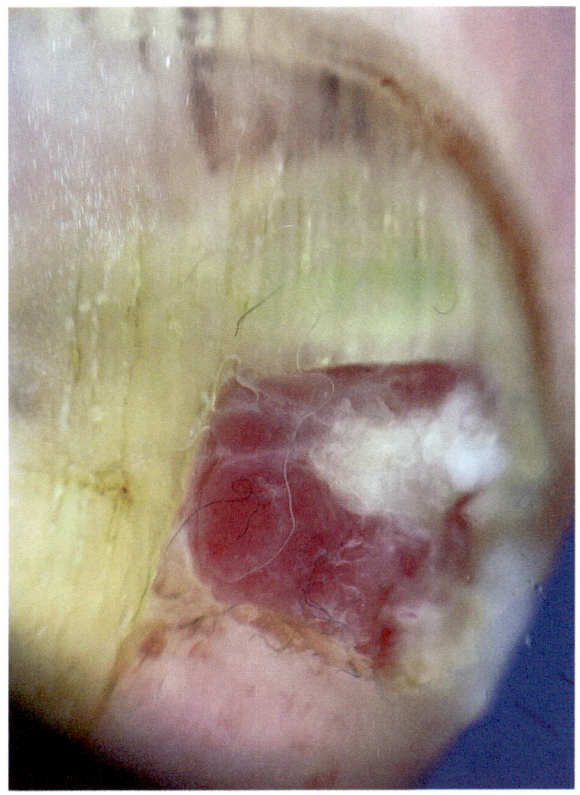

Based on the Case Description and the Photographs? What Is Your Diagnosis?

Subungual pyogenic granuloma—squamous cell carcinoma—amelanotic melanoma

Diagnosis

Subungual epidermoid carcinoma

Discussion

Nail unit squamous cell carcinoma (NUSCC) is the most common nail malignancy with a 2:1 male-to-female ratio, typically occurring after the age of 50. Risk factors include ionizing radiations, tobacco, trauma, arsenic exposure and human papillomavirus (HPV) infection [1] . It is estimated that more than 50% of NUSCC are associated with HPV [2], high-risk types, notably HPV16, responsible for half of the cases of *in situ* variants and almost ¾ of invasive cases [2].

Some authors consider that this is a sexually transmitted disease, as it results from a genital digital contamination and that self inoculation is responsible for polydactylic forms [2].

The evolution is very slow and delay to diagnosis is usually between 2 to 5 years [3]. Immunosuppressed patients are more prone to develop NUSCC, especially HPV16 linked, at an earlier age. Polydactylic forms are more common in this group [4].

There are two main clinical presentations, both occurring at the same frequency [2]:

1. A periungual form, verrucous, mostly misdiagnosed as a wart.
2. A nodular subungal form developing from the bed, with subsequent oozing and onycholysis.

The association of a longitudinal melanonychia on the lateral side of the plate is strongly linked with HPV56 infection and amazingly these lesions have been shown to be always *in situ* [2].

Nail dermoscopy is rarely useful in the periungual variant as it will only show a verrucous aspect. The subungual form shows dermatoscopic features observed elsewhere on the body (clusters of dot-like to glomerular vessels, milky-red areas …).

Radiologic evaluation, particularly MRI, can assess the deep margin of the tumor and rule out bone invasion and may help to biopsy the best place [5]. About 16% of patients may exhibit bony invasion [6]. However, some studies have shown the unreliability of medical imaging for bone invasion [7, 8]. Histopathology remains the gold standard for diagnosis, although biopsies may not adequately sample the deep margin. Histologic diagnosis is based on epithelial disorganization, atypias, mitotic figures and dyskeratosis [9]. In the bed, the tumour is poorly differentiated and with a greater Breslow compared to the periungual form [10]. In a recent study [11], two types of NSCC have been highlighted: a blue basaloid one, HPV-related characterized by koilocytosis, more likely *in situ*, found in periungual lesions and a pink keratinizing one, non-HPV-related and invasive, found in subungual lesions.

Treatment modalities for NUSCC rely on functional surgery achieving cleared histological margins. Mohs' micrographic surgery and wide local excision are associated with low recurrence rates, regardless of degree of invasion [12]. Mohs micrographic surgery at the nail unit is difficult due to the complex structure of the nail unit. Wide local excision with full-thickness skin graft repair or secondary intention healing is easy and gives excellent cosmetic outcomes [1].

If histology shows bone involvement, amputation is required.

Radiation therapy is an option for patients who are not eligible or decline surgery. Non-surgical alternatives such as cryotherapy, topical agents (5-FU, imiquimod), and photodynamic therapy are less commonly used due to concerns about reaching affected areas adequately and achieving full clearance without histological assessment. HPV vaccination, targeting high-risk HPV types—but not all types of

Fig. 28.3 Immediate post operative aspect after full thickness graft. All margins were clear

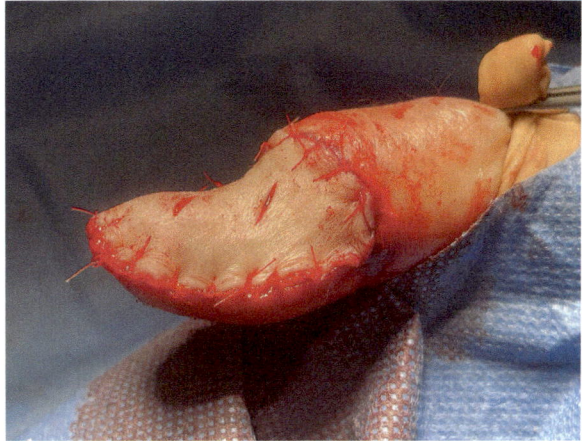

HPV associated NUSCC—may induced in some instances a full tumor regression [13]. HPV vaccination can be an adjuvant therapy, reducing recurrence rates, particularly in cases where surgery may not be feasible or desirable.The systematic vaccination should reduce the number of HPV-induced-NUSCC in the coming years. Prognosis is excellent even in case of invasive forms. Metastases are exceptional.

Our patient, underwent total removal of the nail unit with histology showing cleared margins. The defect was closed by a full thickness graft (Fig. 28.3). A biannual follow-up was set up.

Key Points

- NUSCC is underdiagnosed from its polymorphous clinical features and the reluctance of physicians to biopsy.
- Main cause is high-risk oncogenic HPV
- Bone involvement should be evaluated on histology as medical imaging may give false information
- Treatment relies on functional surgery (= removal of the tumour with cleared margins). Amputation is restricted on proven bony involvement on histology.

References

1. Lecerf P, Richert B, Theunis A, André J. A retrospective study of squamous cell carcinoma of the nail unit diagnosed in a Belgian general hospital over a 15 year period. J Am Acad Dermatol. 2013 Aug;69:253–61.
2. Shimizu A, Kuriyama Y, Hasegawa M, Tamura A, Ishikawa O. Nail squamous cell carcinoma: a hidden high-risk human papillomavirus reservoir for sexually transmitted infections. J Am Acad Dermatol. 2019;81:1358–70.

3. Dijksterhuis A, Friedeman E, van der Heijden B. Squamous cell carcinoma of the nail unit: review of the literature. J Hand Surg Am. 2018;43:374–379.e2.
4. Ormerod E, de Berker D. Nail unit squamous cell carcinoma in people with immunosuppression. Br J Dermatol. 2015;173:701–12.
5. Ammar A, Salon A, Moulonguet I, Drapé JL. MRI of squamous cell carcinoma of the nail apparatus: report of 6 cases. Skeletal Radiol. 2023;52:613–22.
6. Clark MA, Filitis D, Samie FH, Piliang M, Knackstedt TJ. Evaluating the utility of routine imaging in squamous cell carcinoma of the nail unit. Dermatologic Surg. 2020;46:1375–81.
7. Stiff KM, Jellinek N, Knackstedt TJ. A call for evidence-based conservative management of nail unit malignancies. Plast Reconstr Surg. 2022;149:720e–30e.
8. Dika E, Piraccini BM, Balestri R, Vaccari S, Misciali C, Patrizi A, Fanti PA. Mohs surgery for squamous cell carcinoma of the nail: report of 15 cases. Our experience and a long-term follow-up. Br J Dermatol. 2012;167:1310–4.
9. André J, Sass U, Theunis A. Diseases of the nails. In: Calonje E, Brenn T, Lazar AJ, Billings SD, editors. McKee's pathology of the skin with clinical correlations. 5th ed. Elsevier; 2020. p. 1129–555.
10. Dika E, de Biase D, Lambertini M, Alessandrini AM, Acquaviva G, De Leo A, Tallini G, Ricci C, Starace M, Misciali C, Piraccini BM. Mutational landscape in squamous cell carcinoma of the nail unit. Exp Dermatol. 2022;31:854–61.
11. Moulart F, Olemans C, De Saint Aubain N, Richert B, André J. Squamous Cell Carcinoma of the Nail Apparatus: Histopathology and Immunohistochemistry Correlation Study. J Cutaneous Pathol, accepted for publication.
12. Ning AY, Levoska MA, Zheng DX, Carroll BT, Wong CY. Treatment options and outcomes for squamous cell carcinoma of the nail unit: a systematic review. Dermatologic Surg. 2022;48:267–73.
13. Jeon YJ, Koo DW, Lee JS. Bowen disease of the nail apparatus with HPV16 positivity and resolution with human papillomavirus vaccination. Br J Dermatol. 2020;183:e1.

Chapter 29
Nail Dystrophy and Lymphedema

Kimberly M. Ken (iD) **and Adam I. Rubin** (iD)

Abstract Yellow Nail Syndrome (YNS) is characterized by the triad of yellow nails, respiratory manifestations, and lymphedema. Nail changes can affect both fingers and toes and consist primarily of xanthonychia, thickened nail plates, transverse over-curvature, onycholysis and slow to absent growth. Treatment for YNS, which most often includes systemic Vitamin E with or without oral fluconazole, is aimed at improving the appearance of the nails and any associated discomfort.

Keywords Yellow nails · Xanthonychia · Lymphedema · Bronchiectasis · Sinusitis

Clinical Case

A 76-year-old male presented to clinic with a 2-year history of abnormal finger and toenails that were yellow in coloration, thickened, and with distal onycholysis (Fig. 29.1). Recently, he developed bilateral lower extremity lymphedema. During his lymphedema evaluation, he was found to have pleural effusions and bronchiectasis. He has a history of sinusitis and underwent surgery for a deviated septum 4 years ago.

K. M. Ken (✉)
Department of Dermatology, Penn State Health and Penn State College of Medicine, Hershey, PA, USA
e-mail: kken@pennstatehealth.psu.edu

A. I. Rubin
Ronald O. Perelman Department of Dermatology, New York University Grossman School of Medicine, New York, NY, USA
e-mail: Adam.Rubin@nyulangone.org

© The Author(s), under exclusive license to Springer Nature   169
Switzerland AG 2025
A. Tosti et al. (eds.), *Clinical Cases in Nail Disorders*, Clinical Cases in
Dermatology, https://doi.org/10.1007/978-3-031-88642-3_29

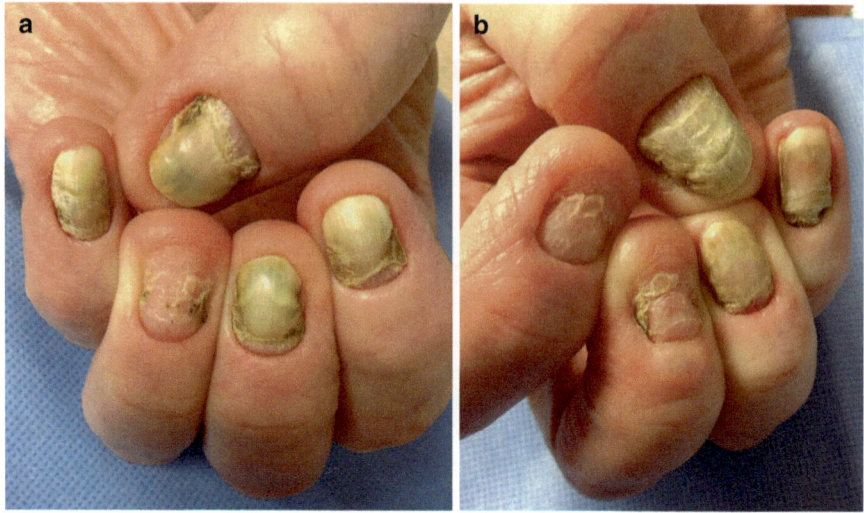

Fig. 29.1 Nail dystrophy at time of presentation. (**a**) Left hand. (**b**) Right hand. (Credit: Adam Rubin, MD)

What Is Your Diagnosis?

Yellow Nail Syndrome (YNS)
Shell nail syndrome
Digital Clubbing
Nail Lichen Planus

Diagnosis

Yellow Nail Syndrome

Discussion

Overview and Presentation

Yellow Nail Syndrome (YNS), first described by Samman and White in 1964, is a rare disorder characterized by the triad of yellow nails, respiratory manifestations, and lymphedema with two out of three required for diagnosis [1–3]. Nails are yellow, very hard, and have slow or absent growth. Chronic paronychia and onycholysis may be seen [3].

Lymphedema, thought to be secondary to lymphatic dysfunction, is seen in 30–80% of cases and most often involves the lower extremities [3, 4]. Pulmonary manifestations vary from chronic cough, most frequently, to pleural effusions and recurrent pulmonary infections [3, 5]. Acute or chronic sinusitis occurs commonly in YNS affecting between 14–83% of cases [3]. The etiology of YNS is not fully understood, but thought to be related to dysfunction in lymphatic drainage. There have been associations of YNS with malignancy, immunodeficiencies, and autoimmune disorders [6].

Treatment

YNS may resolve spontaneously, can improve with treatment of underlying respiratory disorders, and, if paraneoplastic, there are reports of resolution when the underlying malignancy is treated [3, 5]. The goal for YNS treatment is to improve the appearance of the nails and any associated discomfort, if onycholysis or chronic paronychia exist. Given the rarity of YNS, there is not a standard therapy however the most reported treatments include systemic Vitamin E, with or without oral fluconazole, and oral clarithromycin [3, 4, 7] The patient in this case was initially treated with intralesional nail matrix triamcinolone 5 mg/mL injections every 2–4 months and systemic vitamin E (initially 800 IU and then 1200 IU daily) with some improvement in his nails (Fig. 29.2). Around one year into treatment, he was started on oral fluconazole 300 mg weekly and continued oral vitamin E and intralesional triamcinolone to the affected nails and had great improvement in the majority of his nails. Any recalcitrant nails were then treated with intralesional triamcinolone 7.5 mg/mL with continued improvement (Fig. 29.3). He has almost normal nails and has been on treatment for around 5 years.

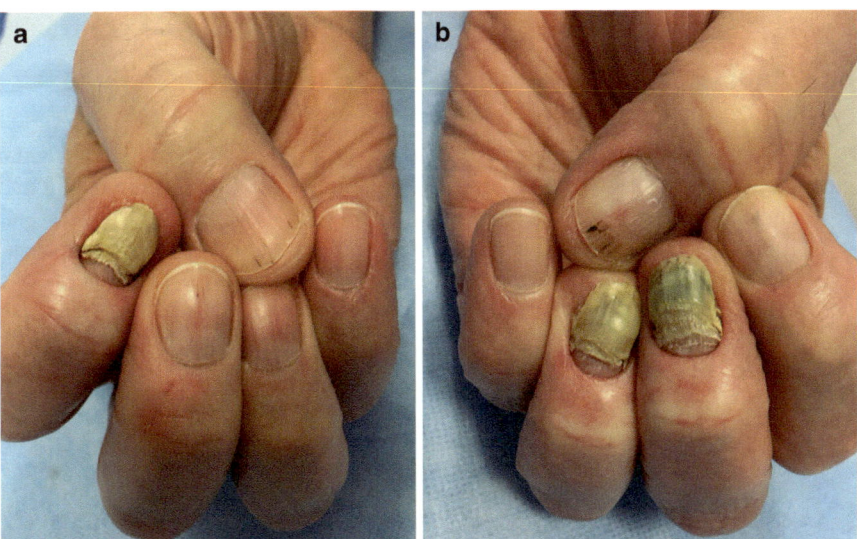

Fig. 29.2 Improvement in YNS after 1 year of treatment with oral Vitamin E, oral fluconazole and intralesional triamcinolone. (**a**) Right hand. (**b**) Left hand. (Credit: Adam Rubin, MD)

Fig. 29.3 Almost complete resolution of YNS following 3 years of treatment including oral Vitamin E, oral fluconazole and intralesional triamcinolone. (Credit: Adam Rubin, MD)

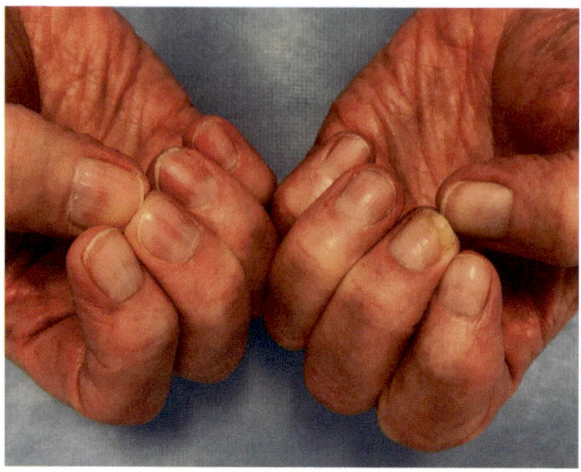

Review of Differential Diagnosis

Although digital clubbing can be associated with bronchiectasis and pulmonary infections, the clinical findings are distinct from YNS with hypertrophy of the distal digital soft tissue and bidirectional increase in the diameter of the nail plate [8, 9]. Shell nail syndrome is also associated with bronchiectasis and has similar features to digital clubbing, but the distal nail bed in shell nails is atrophic [9]. Nail lichen planus can present with a slight yellowish coloration of the nails, however this is often accompanied by nail plate thinning, longitudinal ridging, and dorsal pterygium which were not seen in this patient.

Key Points

- Yellow nail syndrome is characterized by the triad of yellow nails, lymphedema, and respiratory disorders. A diagnosis requires 2 of the 3 aforementioned findings.
- Nail changes can affect fingers and/or toes and consist of xanthonychia, thickened nail plates, transverse over-curvature, onycholysis and slow to absent growth.

References

1. Samman PD, White WF. The "yellow nail" syndrome. Br J Dermatol. 1964;76:153–7. https://doi.org/10.1111/j.1365-2133.1964.tb14499.x.
2. Maldonado F, Ryu JH. Yellow nail syndrome. Curr Opin Pulm Med. 2009;15(4):371–5. https://doi.org/10.1097/MCP.0b013e32832ad45a.

3. Vignes S, Baran R. Yellow nail syndrome: a review. Orphanet J Rare Dis. 2017;12(1):42. https://doi.org/10.1186/s13023-017-0594-4.

4. Benassaia E, Abba S, Fourgeaud C, Mihoubi A, Vignes S. Yellow nail syndrome: analysis of 23 consecutive patients and effect of combined fluconazole-vitamin-E treatment. Dermatology. 2023;240:343–51. https://doi.org/10.1159/000535577.

5. Maldonado F, Tazelaar HD, Wang CW, Ryu JH. Yellow nail syndrome: analysis of 41 consecutive patients. Chest. 2008;134(2):375–81. https://doi.org/10.1378/chest.08-0137.

6. Schneider SL, Tosti A. Tips to diagnose uncommon nail disorders. Dermatol Clin. 2015;33(2):197–205. https://doi.org/10.1016/j.det.2014.12.003.

7. Matsubayashi S, Suzuki M, Suzuki T, et al. Effectiveness of clarithromycin in patients with yellow nail syndrome. BMC Pulm Med. 2018;18(1):138. https://doi.org/10.1186/s12890-018-0707-4.

8. Sarkar M, Mahesh DM, Madabhavi I. Digital clubbing. Lung India. 2012;29(4):354–62. https://doi.org/10.4103/0970-2113.102824.

9. Zaiac MN, Walker A. Nail abnormalities associated with systemic pathologies. Clin Dermatol. 2013;31(5):627–49. https://doi.org/10.1016/j.clindermatol.2013.06.018.

Chapter 30
Pediatric Nail Matrix Nevus: Diagnostic Challenges and Management Strategies

Bengü Nisa Akay ⓘ, **Ece Gökyayla** ⓘ, **Mustafa Turhan Şahin** ⓘ, **and Luc Thomas**

Abstract The presence of longitudinal melanonychia in a single nail of a child poses a diagnostic challenge for clinicians, as worrisome dermatoscopic features of nail matrix melanoma are commonly found in childhood nevi. Luckily, matrix melanoma is exceptionally rare in this age group.

Keywords Pediatric nail matrix nevi · Adult nail matrix melanoma · Dermoscopic features

Clinical Cases

Patient 1

The first case involved a 6-year-old girl with pigmentation appearing on her right thumb nail approximately 3 months prior to her presentation (Fig. 30.1). The patient was monitored periodically, and within 2 years, the pigmentation had extended to cover almost the entire nail (Fig. 30.2).

B. N. Akay
Faculty of Medicine, Department of Dermatology and Venereology, Ankara University, Ankara, Türkiye

E. Gökyayla
Department of Dermatology and Venereology, Uşak Training and Research Hospital, Uşak, Türkiye

M. T. Şahin (✉)
Faculty of Medicine, Department of Dermatology and Venereology, Manisa Celal Bayar University, Manisa, Türkiye

L. Thomas
Hospices Civils de Lyon 1 University, Lyon, France
e-mail: luc.thomas@chu-lyon.fr

Differential diagnosis:

- Subungual hemorrhage
- Nail matrix nevus
- Malignant melanoma
- Melanotic macule of nail unit

Correct diagnosis is nail matrix nevus. This consistent progression suggests a congenital type of nail unit involvement. Choosing not to perform a biopsy was based on several factors. Firstly, if a biopsy was conducted, continued follow-up would be necessary. Additionally, complete excision of the nail matrix nevus could result in severe dystrophy, which would be a significant outcome for a thumb and would not eliminate the need for ongoing follow-up, as recurrent pigmentation could complicate management. Furthermore, complete excision of the nail unit along with grafting would lead to definitive anonychia and potential disability for the child's entire life. Given the patient's age of 6 years and the likelihood of at least partial regression of the lesion after puberty, follow-up was deemed the most appropriate management approach.

Patient 2

The second patient, a 2-year-old baby boy, presented with a rapidly growing pigmented lesion on the left thumb nail, with a duration of 3 months (Fig. 30.3). Initially, the only suspicious dermatoscopic findings were triangular longitudinal

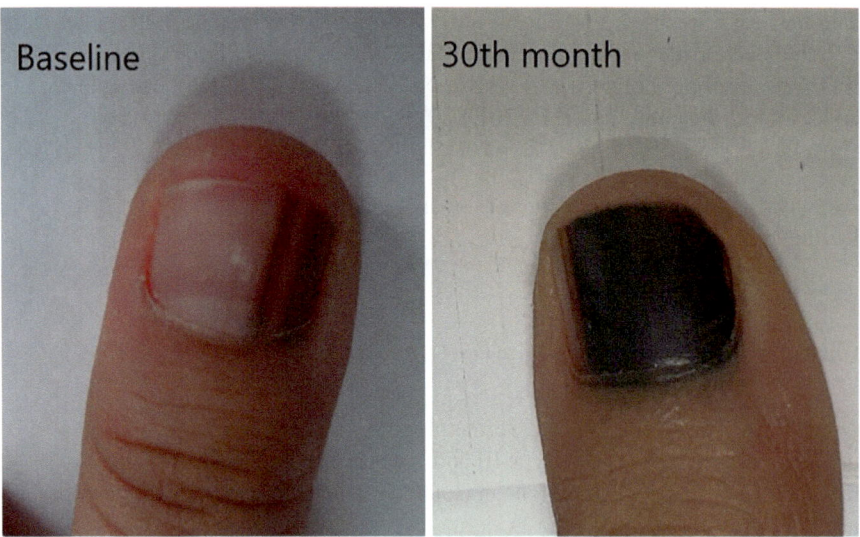

Fig. 30.1 Clinical Appearance of the Right Thumb Nail: Baseline and 30-month follow-up in a 6-year-old girl. In the second photo, pigmentation is observed to have extended to nearly the entire nail

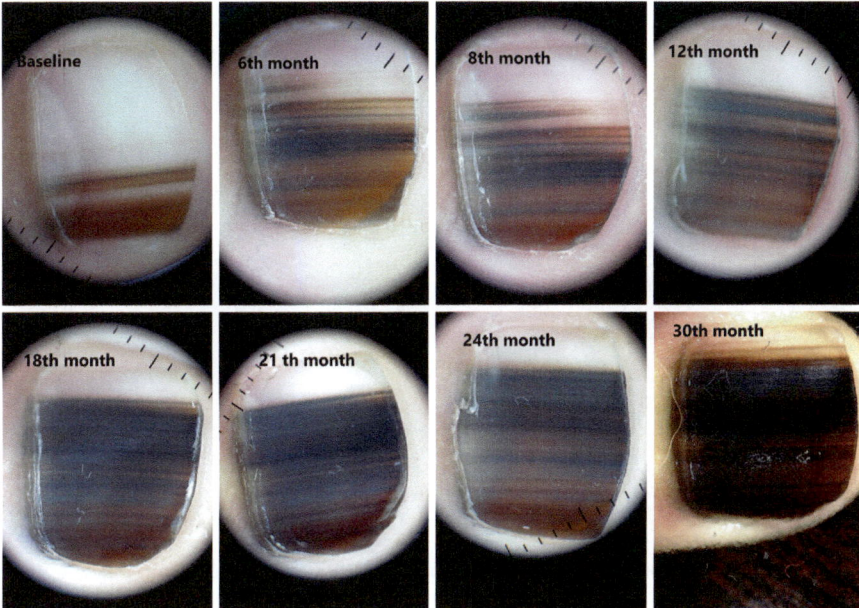

Fig. 30.2 Dermatoscopic Progression Over Time. Dermatoscopic views from baseline to the 30th month are compared. The pigmentation, initially light brown and covering 1/3 of the nail in the baseline photograph, progressed to a very dark brown-black pigmentation, nearly covering the entire nail by the 30th month. Pigmented bands exhibited irregularities during follow-up, with variations in width, interval, and colors

melanonychia and pigmented bands varying in width and intervals, features commonly seen in pediatric nail matrix nevi. However, over the following 3 months, the lesion rapidly expanded, with pigmented bands covering almost the entire nail (Fig. 30.4). Additional atypical dermatoscopic findings, such as nail fissuring, bleeding, and periungual pigmentation, emerged, prompting a biopsy of the lesion, which was performed by the Plastic Surgery department.

Differential diagnosis:

- Subungual hemorrhage
- Nail matrix nevus
- Malignant melanoma
- Melanotic macule of nail unit

Pathology results indicated a congenital nail matrix nevus. Despite the Plastic Surgeon performing a matricectomy, the nail regrew 4 months later, appearing dystrophic and highly pigmented (Fig. 30.5). Regrettably, we are compelled to continue monitoring the patient in this manner. Given the rarity of nail matrix melanomas in the pediatric period, maintaining a high biopsy threshold is essential. Follow-up remains the optimal approach in this case.

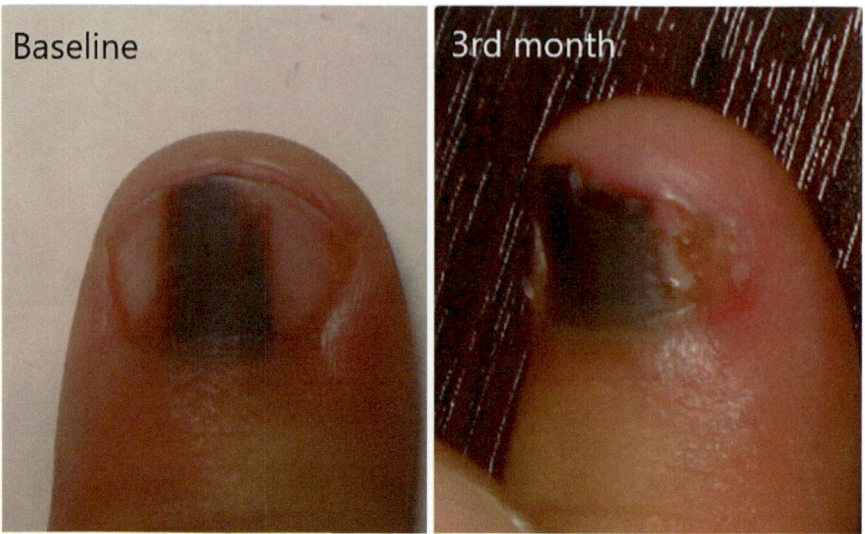

Fig. 30.3 Clinical Appearance of the Left Thumb Nail: Baseline and 3-month follow-up in a 2 year-old baby boy. In the second photo, pigmentation is observed to have extended to nearly the entire nail and an accompanied paronychia

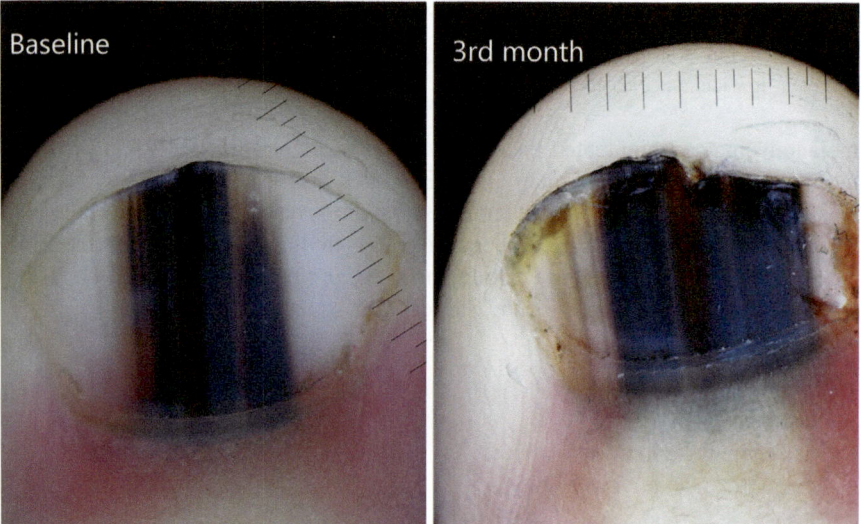

Fig. 30.4 Baseline Dermatoscopy shows triangular longitudinal melanonychia, along with variations in the width, interval, and coloration of the pigmented bands, are observed. Third Month Dermatoscopy. Pigmentation has extended to nearly the entire nail. Additionally, features such as a fissuring at the nail tip, lateral bleeding, pseudohutchinson sign, and also mild pigmentation on the proximal nail skin are observed

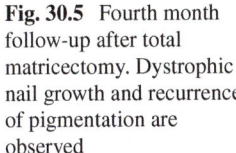

Fig. 30.5 Fourth month follow-up after total matricectomy. Dystrophic nail growth and recurrence of pigmentation are observed

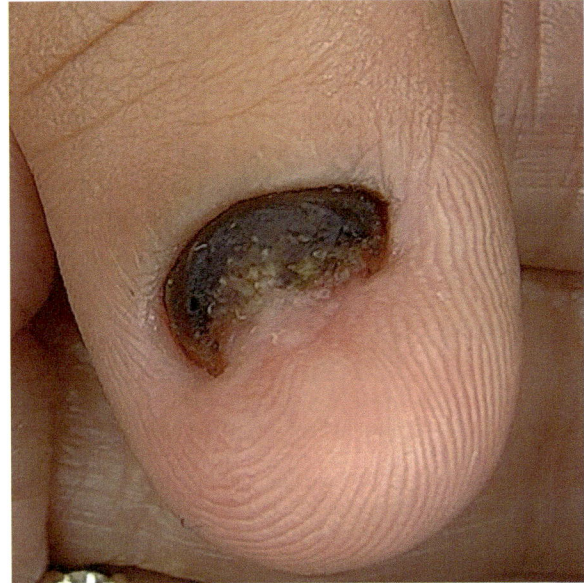

Discussion

The presence of longitudinal melanonychia in a single nail of a child poses a diagnostic challenge for clinicians, as worrisome dermatoscopic features of nail matrix melanoma are commonly found in childhood nevi. Nail matrix melanoma is exceptionally rare in this age group. [1, 2]

Previously reported cases of pediatric nail unit melanoma [3] have been considered by some authors as atypical, likely representing benign lentiginous melanocytic hyperplasia or highly active junctional nevi rather than melanoma [4]. Subsequently, other reports described acral melanomas in children, supported by evidence from immunohistochemical staining (p16, S-100, HMB-45). Despite its rarity, nail matrix melanoma in children can progress rapidly and display concerning clinical and dermatoscopic features [1, 2].

Dermatoscopic features commonly associated with melanoma in adults, such as pigmented lines varying in width, interval, and color, disruption of parallelism, triangular-shaped bands, blurred lateral borders, pigmentation of the periungual skin, and nail plate fissuring or splitting, are also frequently found in childhood subungual nevi due to activation of nail matrix melanocytes [5]. Consequently, these features are not considered reliable indicators for biopsy, although there is ongoing debate in the literature.

Management involves careful observation, with biopsy reserved for cases showing atypical features or rapid growth. Invasive procedures carry risks of severe outcomes, emphasizing the importance of follow-up and consideration of the child's age and potential for lesion regression.

Key Points

Here, we present two cases of pediatric nail matrix nevi exhibiting findings similar to those of adult nail matrix melanomas, highlighting the diagnostic challenges they pose. We discuss the approach to managing such cases, emphasizing the importance of careful observation and consideration of atypical features or rapid progression, given the potential severity of outcomes associated with invasive procedures.

References

1. Bonamonte D, Arpaia N, Cimmino A, et al. In situ melanoma of the nail unit presenting as a rapid growing longitudinal melanonychia in a 9-year-old white boy. Dermatologic Surg. 2014;40:1154–7.
2. Iorizzo M, Tosti A, Di Chiacchio N, et al. Nail melanoma in children: differential diagnosis and management. Dermatologic Surg. 2008;34:974–8.
3. Kato T, Usuba Y, Takematsu H, et al. A rapidly growing pigmented nail streak resulting in diffuse melanosis of the nail. A possible sign of subungual melanoma in situ. Cancer. 1989;64:2191–7.
4. Goettmann-Bonvallot S, Andre J, Belaich S. Longitudinal melanonychia in children: a clinical and histopathologic study of 40 cases. J Am Acad Dermatol. 1999;41:17–22.
5. Pham F, Boespflug A, Duru G, Phan A, et al. Dermatoscopic and clinical features of congenital or congenital-type nail matrix nevi: a multicenter prospective cohort study by the international Dermoscopy society. J Am Acad Dermatol. 2022;87:551–8.

Chapter 31
Acquired Pincer Nail Deformity of the Right Thumb

Andrea Sechi and Anna Bolzon

Abstract Background: Pincer nail deformity is marked by abnormal curvature of the nail plate, often causing discomfort and pain. It is commonly reported in toenails and rarely in fingernails, where it can indicate underlying pathology, including subungual tumors.

Case Presentation: A 64-year-old male presented to our service with a 9-month history of acquired pincer nail deformity of the right thumb. Clinical and dermoscopic examination revealed a thickened, yellow-colored, over-curved nail plate with underlying compact hyperkeratosis. High-frequency ultrasound detected a subungual hypoechoic lesion, and an X-ray scan showed osteoarthritic changes without bone erosion. Surgical excision was performed, and showed a polypoid lesion involving the nail matrix and bed, after avulsion of the nail plate. Histopathology examination diagnosed superficial acral fibromyxoma, characterized by spindle cell proliferation in a fibro-myxoid stroma, with CD34 and CD99 immunoreactivity.

Discussion: Superficial acral fibromyxoma is a rare benign tumor affecting the nail unit, and is characterized by protean clinical features, including a subungual whitish or pinkish mass distorting the nail plate, pincer nail deformity or pterygium-like aspect.

Imaging and histopathology are mandatory to achieve the correct diagnosis, distinguishing it from malignant myxoid tumors. Full excision of the lesion is recommended to prevent recurrence.

Conclusion: Isolated pincer nail deformity in a fingernail warrants investigation for potential subungual lesions, including superficial acral fibromyxoma.

A. Sechi (✉)
Dermatology Unit, Fondazione IRCCS Ca' Granda Ospedale Maggiore Policlinico, Milan, Italy

A. Bolzon
Dermatology Unit, Department of Medicine (DIMED), University of Padova, Padova, Italy

Keywords Pincer nail deformity · Superficial acral fibromyxoma ·
Subungual tumor

Case Presentation

A 64-year-old male patient was referred to our nail outpatient service with a 9-month
history of an acquired pincer nail deformity in the right thumb. The patient's medical history was significant for hypertension treated with ACE inhibitors and hyper-
cholesterolemia managed with statins. The patient worked in an office setting and
denied any recent history of trauma; he reported pain upon palpation at the nail plate
and constant discomfort in the lateral and proximal nail folds. The patient also
denied any cold sensitivity.

Clinical Findings

On examination, the nail plate was thickened and opaque with a yellowish discoloration
distal to the lunula (xanthonychia) and exhibited a narrowing of the distal end along the
longitudinal axis, with an increased maximum transverse curvature (Fig. 31.1a, b). The
lateral edges of the nail plate were embedded in the lateral nail folds. There were no
swellings in the distal interphalangeal joint, and the patient did not report joint pain. The
curvature index, defined as the traced length of the nail plate at the tip divided by the
apparent width of the nail tip [1], was 1.8. Onychoscopy revealed longitudinal parallel
white and yellowish lines, longitudinal fissuring of the nail plate, splinter hemorrhages
at the onychodermal band. At the free edge the nail plate was overcurved and thickened,
and was associated with a moderate subungual hyperkeratosis; no glomerular vessels
were detectable at the hyponychium (Fig. 31.2a–d).

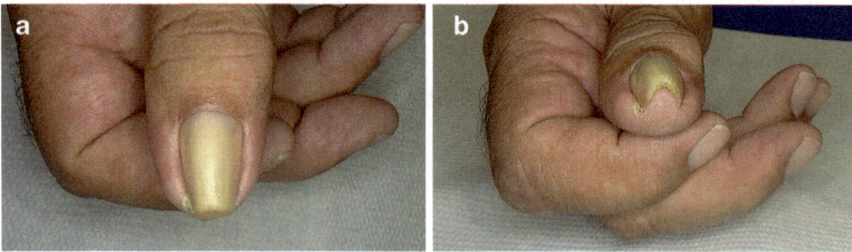

Fig. 31.1 Clinical presentation of the acquired pincer nail deformity of the right thumb. The nail
is characterized by the progressive thickening of the nail plate towards the distal end with a yellowish discoloration (**a**), accompanied by pronounced over-curvature at the free margin and apparent
shrinkage of the nail bed (**b**)

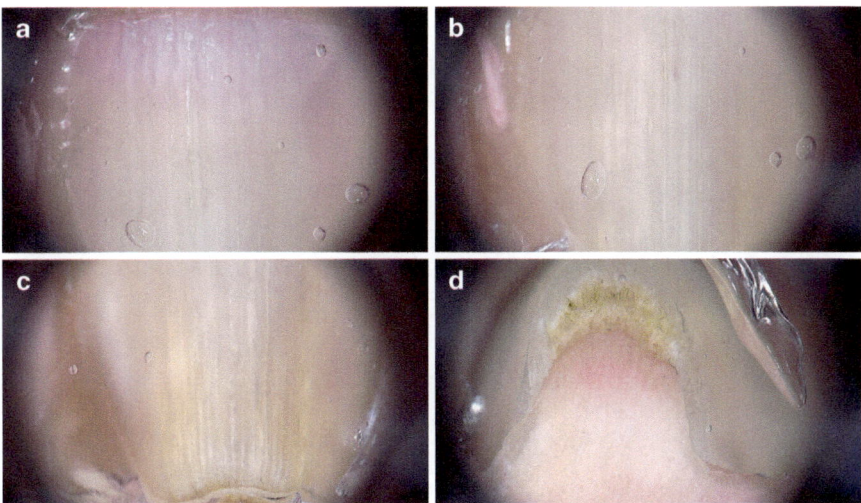

Fig. 31.2 Onychoscopy at 20x magnification displays linear whitish lines originating from the lunula (**a**) and extending longitudinally across the entire nail plate, with associated splinter hemorrhages and longitudinal fissures (**b**). Additional yellowish lines become more detectable at the onychodermal band, possibly due to the increased overcurvature of the nail plate (**c**). Beneath the nail plate at the free margin, subungual hyperkeratosis is present; no enhanced vascularity is evident at the hyponychium (**d**)

Diagnostic Assessment

High-frequency ultrasound performed at 18 MHz (MyLab One, Esaote S.p.A., Genova, Italy) detected a subungual ovoid lobulated hypoechoic formation measuring 11 mm in longitudinal diameter and 4.6 mm in axial diameter, with cup shape remodeling of the underlying phalanx (Fig. 31.3a). X-ray findings showed no sign of bone erosion, osteoarthritic changes in the first digit's distal interphalangeal joint, with reduced joint space, sclerosis of bone margins, and intra-articular calcifications (Fig. 31.3b).

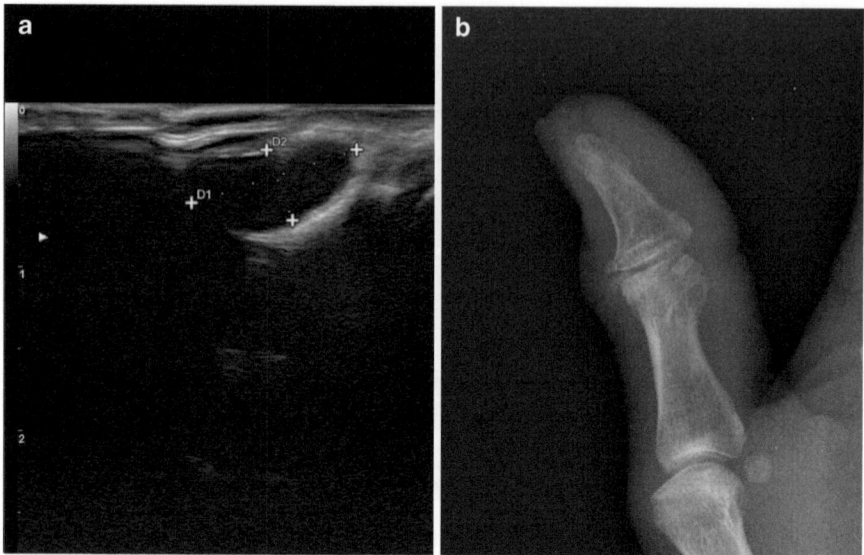

Fig. 31.3 (a) High-frequency ultrasound Greyscale B-mode longitudinal scan showing a well-defined subungual hypo/anechoic lobulated lesion, which causes a cup-shape remodeling of the underlying bone. (b) X-ray film showed osteoarthritic changes of the interphalangeal joint and no sign of bone erosion of the distal phalanx

Workout

During the excision procedure, the proximal nail fold (PNF) was reclined with two lateral incisions. The PNF was then carefully separated from the underlying nail plate using a nail elevator.

The nail plate was detached from the nail bed along a plane of cleavage, and then incised along the lateral margins of the parallel bands of leukoxanthonychia using a straight-tip scissor. This exposed a whitish mass at the lunula and whitish projections along the nail bed and the hyponychium (Fig. 31.4). The mass in the distal matrix was shaved and a longitudinal biopsy was performed to include the nail bed up to the hyponychium. Also, the matrix horns were sectioned and cauterized with 10% NaOH to reduce the width of the nail.

The pathology report revealed a polypoid lesion within the nail matrix, characterized by epidermal hyperplasia and spindle cell proliferation in a fibro-collagenous stroma with prominent vascular features. Reactive atypical features were present, along with numerous mast cells in the dermis.

Specimens from the nail bed showed similar epidermal hyperplasia with spindle cells set in a fibro-myxoid stroma, suggesting a rich vascular network. The nail plate fragments demonstrated epidermal hyperkeratosis. Immunohistochemical staining showed focal positivity for CD34 and CD99, with negativity for S100 and EMA (Fig. 31.5).

Fig. 31.4 Intraoperative view displaying a well-defined ivory-white mass located at the distal matrix, with visible whitish structural changes affecting the nail bed and hyponychium

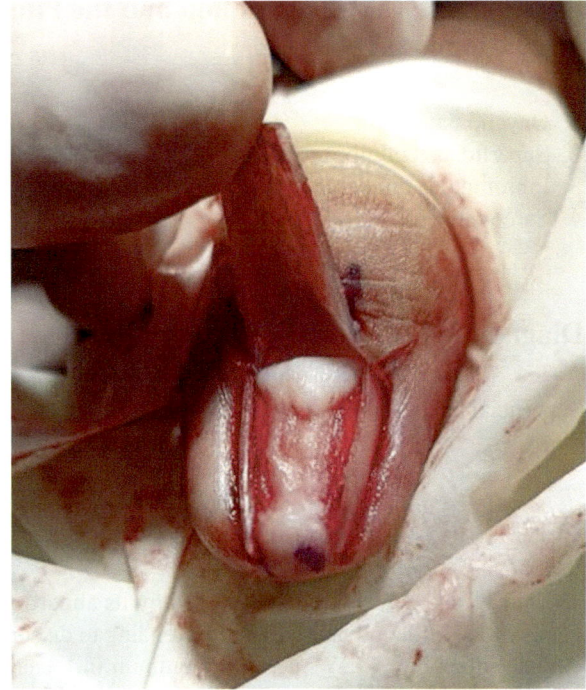

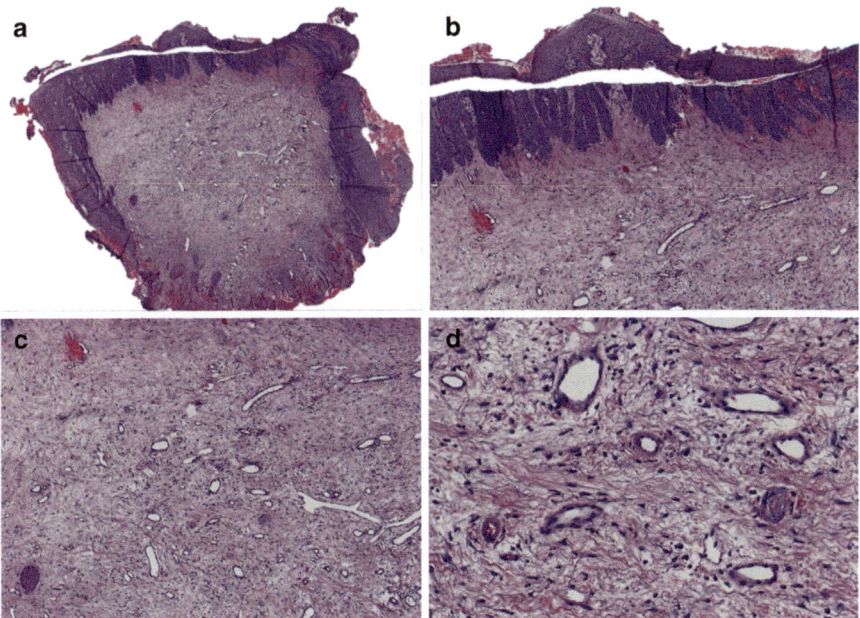

Fig. 31.5 H&E stains at 2× (**a**), 5× (**b**), 10× (**c**), 20× (**d**) magnifications. (Courtesy of Dr. Deborah Saraggi)

Based on the Case Description and the Photographs, What Is Your Diagnosis?

1. Onychomatricoma
2. Superficial acral fibromyxoma
3. Fibromatous tumors
4. Sarcoma

Diagnosis

Superficial acral fibromyxoma

Discussion

The pincer nail deformity is recognized by its abnormally curved nail plate, which compresses the lateral nail folds, often leading to discomfort, pain, and potential for chronic infections [2]. While more common in toenails, especially the great toenails, it can also affect fingernails. The causes of pincer nail deformity are multifactorial, with both genetic and acquired factors implicated. Hereditary cases can present during adolescence or early adulthood, frequently involving multiple nails and following autosomal dominant inheritance patterns [3], such as in Clouston syndrome [4].

Acquired pincer nail deformity is associated with various systemic diseases including gastrointestinal malignancies, renal failure [5], and systemic lupus erythematosus [2]. Some cases may resolve with the treatment of the underlying disease. Pincer nail can also result from local factors, such as pressure from tight shoes, trauma, nail avulsion, or infections like tinea unguium [6, 7]. Certain medications, including beta-blockers and pamidronate, have been known to induce pincer nails, which may reverse after discontinuing the drugs [8].

When a pincer nail is confined to a single digit, particularly a fingernail, the possibility of a nail tumor should be considered. Benign nail tumors, including onychomatricoma [9] and superficial acral fibromyxoma [10] (SAFM), can cause localized or diffuse thickening of the nail plate. Myxoid cysts [11], epidermoid cysts [12], subungual exostosis [13], and osteoarthritis in the distal interphalangeal joints are other potential causes [2].

In the presented case, SAFM was diagnosed. This soft tissue tumor most commonly affects adults and predominantly arises in subungual or periungual areas. Approximately 60% of SAFM cases are asymptomatic and manifest as subungual or periungual pinkish/whitish lesions causing a progressive distortion of the nail apparatus, with consequent swelling due to compression and inflammatory reaction in the nail bed [14].

On pathology, the diagnostic challenge is to distinguish SAFM from malignant myxoid tumors, which may recur or metastasize. SAFM often exhibits positive CD34 and CD99 immunohistochemical staining, with EMA showing variable results [15].

Radiography rarely shows bone erosion [14]; instead, ultrasound may reveal a hypoechoic core with ill-defined borders, surrounded by a hypo/anechoic halo indicative of a myxoid matrix rather than necrosis [16].

Complete surgical excision with close follow-up is crucial for managing SAFM due to high rates of recurrence, especially when positive margins are present. Up to 89% of cases may have positive margins, and recurrences occur in 20–25% of all cases, often tied to previous positive surgical margins [14].

Key Points

- Single-digit fingernail pincer nail deformity may indicate underlying tumors like SAFM, often diagnosed via imaging and histopathology.
- Radiologically, SAFM presents without bone erosion, with ultrasound showing a hypoanechoic lesion due its myxoid content; pathologically, it exhibits spindle cells in a fibro-myxoid stroma.
- Immunohistochemically, SAFM is CD34 and CD99 positive, aiding differentiation from malignant myxoid tumors, and requires complete surgical excision due to a high recurrence risk from positive margins.

References

1. Yabe T. Curvature index of pincer nail. Plast Reconstr Surg Glob Open. 2013;1(7):e49. https://doi.org/10.1097/GOX.0b013e3182a9647a.
2. Huang C, Huang R, Yu M, Guo W, Zhao Y, Li R, Zhu Z. Pincer nail deformity: clinical characteristics, causes, and managements. Biomed Res Int. 2020;2020:2939850. https://doi.org/10.1155/2020/2939850.
3. Chapman RS. Letter: overcurvature of the nails–an inherited disorder. Br J Dermatol. 1973;89(3):317–8. https://doi.org/10.1111/j.1365-2133.
4. Hu YH, Lin YC, Hwu WL, Lee YM. Pincer nail deformity as the main manifestation of Clouston syndrome. Br J Dermatol. 2015;173(2):581–3. https://doi.org/10.1111/bjd.13703.
5. Hernandez C, Deleon D. Acquired pincer nail deformity associated with renal failure. J Clin Aesthet Dermatol. 2011;4(12):43–5. PMID: 22191008.
6. Sano H, Shionoya K, Ogawa R. Foot loading is different in people with and without pincer nails: a case control study. J Foot Ankle Res. 2015;8:43. https://doi.org/10.1186/s13047-015-0100-y.
7. Higashi N. Pincer nail due to tinea unguium. Hifu. 1990;32:40–4.
8. Greiner D, Schöfer H, Milbradt R. Reversible transverse overcurvature of the nails (pincer nails) after treatment with a beta-blocker. J Am Acad Dermatol. 1998;39(3):486–7.
9. Grover C, Yadav S, Gupta R. An uncommon cause of pincer nail. J Cutan Aesthet Surg. 2023;16(2):159–62. https://doi.org/10.4103/JCAS.JCAS_126_22.

10. Starace M, Vezzoni R, Alessandrini A, Bruni F, Baraldi C, Misciali C, Zelin E, Iorizzo M, Piraccini BM. Superficial acral fibromyxoma: clinical, dermoscopic and histological features of a rare nail tumour. J Eur Acad Dermatol Venereol. 2023;37 https://doi.org/10.1111/jdv.19101.
11. de Berker D, Goettman S, Baran R. Subungual myxoid cysts: clinical manifestations and response to therapy. J Am Acad Dermatol. 2002;46(3):394–8. https://doi.org/10.1067/mjd.2002.119652.
12. Baran R, Broutart J-C. Epidermoid cyst of the thumb presenting as pincer nail. J Am Acad Dermatol. 1988;19(1):143–4. https://doi.org/10.1016/s0190-9622(88)80236-6.
13. García Carmona FJ, Pascual Huerta J, Fernández MD. A proposed subungual exostosis clinical classification and treatment plan. J Am Podiatr Med Assoc. 2009;99(6):519–24. https://doi.org/10.7547/0990519.
14. Hollmann TJ, Bovée JV, Fletcher CD. Digital fibromyxoma (superficial acral fibromyxoma): a detailed characterization of 124 cases. Am J Surg Pathol. 2012;36(6):789–98. https://doi.org/10.1097/PAS.0b013e31824a0b83.
15. Fanti PA, Dika E, Piraccini BM, Infusino SD, Baraldi C, Misciali C. Superficial acral fibromyxoma: a clinicopathological and immunohistochemical analysis of 12 cases of a distinctive soft tissue tumor with a predilection for the fingers and toes. G Ital Dermatol Venereol. 2011;146(4):283–7.
16. Sechi A, Wortsman X. High-frequency ultrasound features of periungual superficial acral fibromyxomas. J Cutan Med Surg. 2023 Sep-Oct;27(5):536–8. https://doi.org/10.1177/12034754231188436.

Chapter 32
Photonycholysis Induced by UVA Curing of Acrylic Gel Nail in a Patient Treated with Doxycycline

Andrea Sechi and Giuseppe Cannata

Abstract *Background:* Photonycholysis is a rare dermatological condition characterized by the detachment of the nail plate from the nail bed following ultraviolet (UV) light exposure. We herein report a rare case of photonycholysis induced by the combination of UV-A curing lamps and doxycycline therapy.

Case Presentation: A 40-year-old woman developed painful onycholysis affecting all fingernails 5 days after using an acrylic gel cured under a 9-watt UV-A lamp. The patient had been on a three-week course of doxycycline for perioral dermatitis. Clinical examination revealed sharply demarcated, rounded onycholysis, sparing the lateral edges of the nail plates. The patient was advised to discontinue doxycycline, trim the affected nails, and apply topical methylprednisolone aceponate 0.1% cream. Full recovery was observed after 3 months.

Discussion: Photonycholysis is an uncommon manifestation of drug-induced photosensitivity, particularly linked to tetracyclines such as doxycycline. UV-A exposure may exacerbates phototoxic reactions by generating reactive oxygen species, and damaging mitochondria in keratinocytes. Three distinct patterns of photonycholysis have been described, with type I, characterized by half-moon-shaped detachment, being most consistent with our case.

Conclusion: This case underscores the importance of recognizing UV-curing lamps and photosensitizing drugs,such as doxycycline, as potential triggers for photonycholysis.

Keywords Photonycholysis · Doxycycline-induced photosensitivity · Photosensitivity reactions · Drug-induced phototoxicity · UV curing lamps · Acrylic gel nails · Tetracycline

A. Sechi (✉)
Dermatology Unit, Fondazione IRCCS Ca' Granda Ospedale Maggiore Policlinico, Milan, Italy

G. Cannata
Dermatology Clinic, IRCCS San Raffaele Hospital, Milan, Italy

A. Tosti et al. (eds.), *Clinical Cases in Nail Disorders*, Clinical Cases in Dermatology, https://doi.org/10.1007/978-3-031-88642-3_32

Introduction

Photonycholysis is an atypical dermatological condition where the nail plate detaches from the nail bed after exposure to ultraviolet (UV) light [1]. This report documents a rare incidence of photonycholysis in relation to UV light and doxycycline.

Case Presentation

We present the case of a 40-year-old female patient who experienced painful onycholysis of all fingernails 5 days post-application of an acrylic gel that was cured under a 9-watt UV-A lamp. The patient had been undergoing treatment with 100 mg of doxycycline twice daily for 3 weeks to treat perioral dermatitis. No other medical history or concurrent medication was reported. Notably, prior similar nail treatments had not resulted in adverse effects. However, this episode led to distinctive rounded shaped onycholysis with sharp proximal borders and accompanying pigmentation (Figs. 32.1 and 32.2). The gel's composition included a blend of acrylate monomers, notably Hydroxypropyl Methacrylate and Aliphatic Polyesterurethane Acrylate.

After removing the acrylic nails herself, the patient was advised to trim the affected nail plates. Treatment with a daily application of methylprednisolone

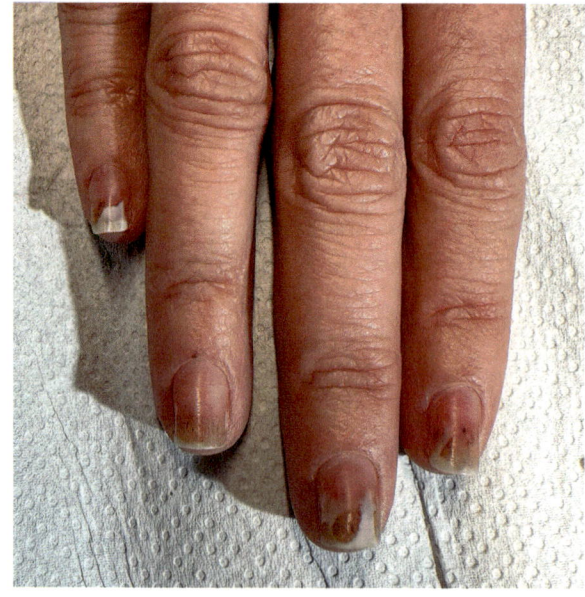

Fig. 32.1 Distal rounded shaped onycholysis with sparing of the lateral aspects of the nail plates, accompanied by surrounding pigmentation. The onycholysis was further exacerbated by the removal of the acrylic gel

Fig. 32.2 Distal onycholysis marked by sharp borders associated with splinter hemorrages of the nail bed

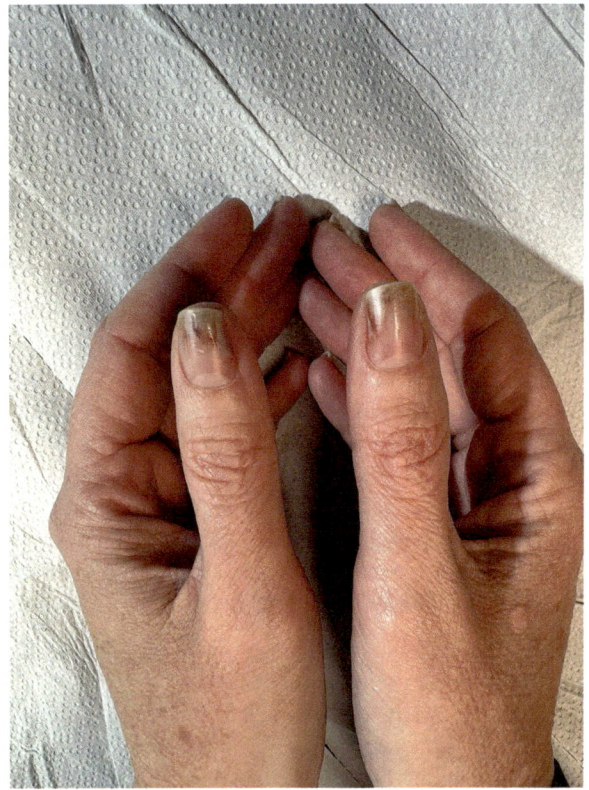

aceponate 0.1% cream facilitated full recovery within 3 months, associated with withdrawal of doxycycline.

Discussion

Although photonycholysis is seldom observed in porphyria, it is also a recognized manifestation of drug-induced photosensitivity, notably associated with tetracyclines, psoralens, and fluoroquinolones [1]. Doxycycline, a tetracycline antibiotic, is documented to precipitate phototoxic reactions that are non-immune mediated and hence restricted to light-exposed skin areas. Such reactions are dose-dependent with respect to both the pharmaceutical and light intensity [2]. The case's UV lamps emitted a spectrum from 300 to 410 nanometers, with peak emission at 375 nanometers [3]. This is supported by studies showing that tetracyclines' phototoxicity may involve singlet oxygen, particularly under UVA radiation [4]. This may cause selective injury to mitochondria, the preferential intracellular site of localization of doxycycline [4]. Moreover, the hierarchy of photo-onycholysis risk among tetracycline variants is established, with doxycycline being significant due to its photoproduct, lumidoxycycline [5]. Furthermore, the typical strategy of administering drugs with shorter half-lives in the evening to minimize phototoxic risk is ineffective for doxycycline. With its longer elimination half-life of 16 to 22 h, doxycycline maintains levels in the system that may lead to phototoxicity at any time of day, regardless of sunlight exposure.

Nail exposure to UV light, which may range between 3% and 20% penetration due to lack of protective melanin, sebum, and the stratum granulosum layer, as well as the convexity of the nail plate acting as a focal lens, are critical factor [1]. Three different patterns of photonycholysis have been reported in the literature [1]:

Type I: characterized by a half-moon-shaped separation of the nail plate that is concave distally. This subtype often exhibits pigmentation of variable intensity with a well-demarcated proximal border.

Type II: exhibits a circular notch opened distally on the nail plate; it is less common and can be identified by a well-defined circular notch with a brownish hue proximally.

Type III: the changes are located in the central part of the nail bed with no connection to the margins. Initially, there may be a round yellow staining that turns reddish after several days. This subtype does not affect the lateral margins of the nails, and the lesion's central positioning is pathognomonic.

In all cases this condition is self-resolving upon discontinuation of the causative drug within 3–6 months.

Interestingly, the clinical manifestation of photonycholysis does not directly correspond with the causative drug. The hallmark of photonycholysis is its distinctive sparing of the nail's lateral edges [6]. Similarly, drug-induced nail alterations can also display a circular pattern, notably when direct damage to blood vessels occurs from chemotherapy agents like taxanes, resulting in subungual haemorrhagic blisters that may progress to onycholysis [7]. Recently, Navarro reported various morphological onycholysis patterns, providing significant diagnostic and therapeutic insights that point to mechanical, chemical, infectious, or systemic disease origins [8]:

- Transversal onycholysis is often linked with trauma or chemical contact, presents as a transverse band of nail detachment;
- Lateral onycholysis is indicative of asymmetric gait nail unit syndrome or subungual lateral onychomycosis, begins from the nail's sides.
- V-shaped onycholysis is suggestive of nail unit tumors or specific conditions like lichen striatus, it is characterized by a V-notch aiming toward the nail's base

Histological examination of photonycholysis reveals mildly dilated blood vessels sans inflammation and a discrete hyperkeratosis, with iron staining returning negative [1].

On dermoscopy, it is characterized by a centrally placed, half-moon-shaped onycholysis with a sharp linear edge, surrounded by red-yellow-brown areas indicative of subungual hemorrhages and hematoma formation on the proximal borders.

Moreover, a "shattered-windshield" pattern characterized by a fragmented nail plate showing a reticular arrangement of white lines has been reported [9].

While cases of photonycholysis following UV curing have not been reported in the past, a novel instance has emerged, detailing photonycholysis manifesting 3 days subsequent to photodynamic therapy utilizing aminolevulinic acid under blue light for the treatment of actinic keratoses [10].

Conclusion

In conclusion, it is critical to acknowledge that light-based devices, including photodynamic therapy and UV curing lamps, may serve as triggers for photonycholysis. This recognition necessitates stringent evaluation and precautionary measures during dermatological procedures involving such devices, particularly for patients with a history of photosensitizing medication use.

Key Points

- Photonycholysis is a rare condition characterized by nail plate detachment from the nail bed, triggered by UV light exposure and exacerbated by photosensitizing drugs like doxycycline.
- The phototoxic reaction originates from UV-A exposure generating reactive oxygen species, causing mitochondrial damage in keratinocytes, with the convex nail plate enhancing UV penetration.
- Photonycholysis presents in patterns such as half-moon-shaped distal detachment (Type I), circular notches (Type II), and central detachment without lateral involvement (Type III).
- Awareness of UV-curing devices and photosensitizing drugs as potential triggers is essential during cosmetic and dermatological treatments to prevent photonycholysis.

References

1. Baran R, Juhlin L. Drug-induced photo-onycholysis. Three subtypes identified in a study of 15 cases. J Am Acad Dermatol. 1987;17(6):1012–6.
2. Hofmann GA, Weber B. Drug-induced photosensitivity: culprit drugs, potential mechanisms and clinical consequences. J Dtsch Dermatol Ges gennaio. 2021;19(1):19–29.
3. Słabicka-Jakubczyk A, Lewandowski M, Pastuszak P, Barańska-Rybak W, Górska-Ponikowska M. Influence of UV nail lamps radiation on human keratinocytes viability. Sci Rep. 2023;13(1):22530.

4. Hasan T, Kochevar IE, McAuliffe DJ, Cooperman BS, Abdulah D. Mechanism of tetracycline phototoxicity. J Invest Dermatol settembre. 1984;83(3):179–83.
5. Al-Kathiri L, Al-Asmaili A. Diclofenac-induced photo-onycholysis. Oman Med J gennaio. 2016;31(1):65–8.
6. Piraccini BM. Drug-induced nail disorders. In: Baran R, De Berker D, Holzberg M, Piraccini BM, Richert B, Thomas L, editors. Baran & Dawber's, diseases of the nails and their management. London: Wiley; 2019. p. 574–603.
7. Alessandrini A, Starace M, Cerè G, Brandi N, Piraccini BM. Management and outcome of taxane-induced nail side effects: experience of 79 patients from a single centre. Skin Appendage Disord agosto. 2019;5(5):276–82.
8. Navarro L. Pattern diagnosis of onycholysis. JEADV Clin Pract. 2023;2(2):213–24.
9. Grover C, Jakhar D. "Shattered-windshield" appearance on dermoscopy in type 1 photo-onycholysis. Indian Dermatol Online J. 2023;14(6):927–8.
10. Paci K, Bell RT, Goldstein B. Fingernail photo-onycholysis after aminolevulinic acid-photodynamic therapy under blue light for treatment of actinic keratoses on the face. Cutis agosto. 2016;98(2):E10–1.

Chapter 33
A Subungual Onycholemmal Cyst Presenting as a Pigmented Band

Katrice M. Karanfilian ⓘ, Daniel Lozeau ⓘ, and Jordan B. Slutsky

Abstract A 52-year-old man presented with a pigmented band on his left great toenail that had been present for three years. As there was concern for melanoma, a nail biopsy was performed resulting in the diagnosis of a subungual onycholemmal cyst. Subungual onycholemmal cysts are rare, benign nail bed neoplasms. They have a variable clinical presentation and definitive diagnosis is made through a nail bed or nail matrix biopsy. On pathology, hyperkeratosis and acanthosis may be present with numerous keratin-filled cysts in the dermis. As this entity is benign, no treatment is necessary although an elective excision may be performed if the lesion is symptomatic. It is important to be aware of the wide range of clinical presentations of subungual onycholemmal cysts and to keep it on the differential diagnosis in patients presenting with a pigmented band on their nail.

Keywords Subungual onycholemmal cyst · Subungual epidermoid cyst · Nail bed · Nail tumor · Pigmented band

K. M. Karanfilian (✉) · J. B. Slutsky
Department of Dermatology, Stony Brook University Hospital, Stony Brook, NY, USA

D. Lozeau
Departments of Dermatology and Pathology, Stony Brook University Hospital,
Stony Brook, NY, USA

© The Author(s), under exclusive license to Springer Nature
Switzerland AG 2025
A. Tosti et al. (eds.), *Clinical Cases in Nail Disorders*, Clinical Cases in
Dermatology, https://doi.org/10.1007/978-3-031-88642-3_33

Clinical Case

A 52-year-old man with asthma, obstructive sleep apnea, hyperlipidemia, and a history of prostate cancer initially presented to the dermatology clinic for discoloration of his left great toenail for three years (Fig. 33.1). He denied any preceding trauma or associated symptoms. Podiatry had treated him previously for suspected onychomycosis with topical antifungal medications and oral terbinafine without success. On physical examination, there was yellow discoloration of the distal aspect of his left great toenail along with a 3-mm central subtle pigment band without Hutchinson's sign. The patient was initially given oral fluconazole 150 mg once weekly and a photograph was taken of the nail for monitoring. At that time, it was thought that the pigment band may be secondary to trauma. After three months, the nail had worsened despite fluconazole. A nail clipping was performed to rule out fungus. As no fungus was revealed, the patient underwent a nail biopsy to rule out melanoma (Fig. 33.2). Pathology revealed multiple keratin-filled cysts in the dermis lined with squamous epithelium lacking a granular layer (Figs. 33.3, 33.4 and 33.5).

Fig. 33.1 Left great toenail at initial presentation

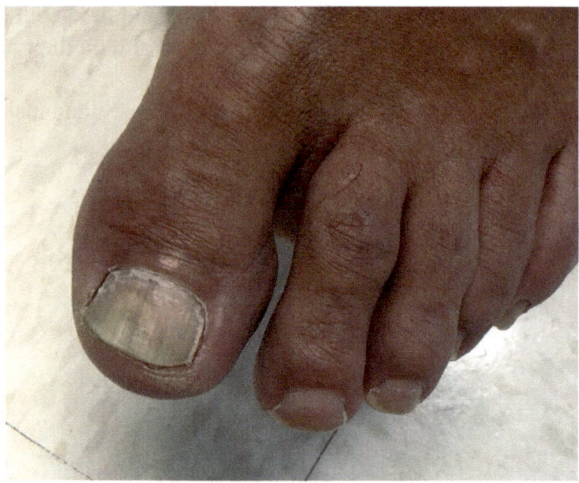

Fig. 33.2 Left great
toenail pre-operatively
prior to nail biopsy

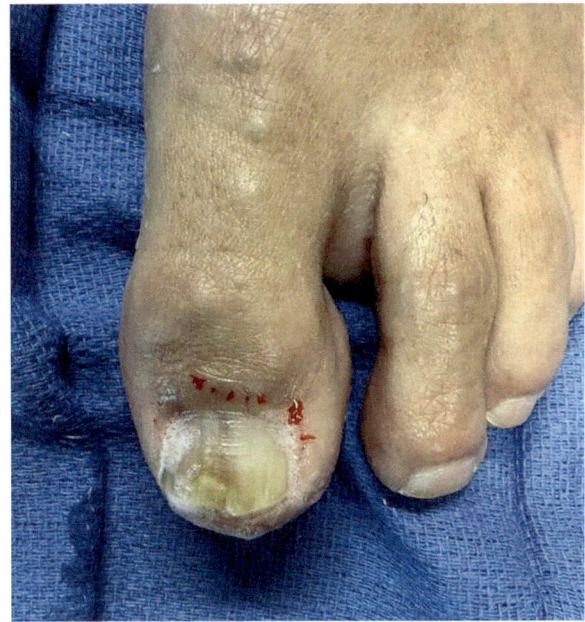

Fig. 33.3 Numerous
keratin-filled cysts in the
dermis, low-power

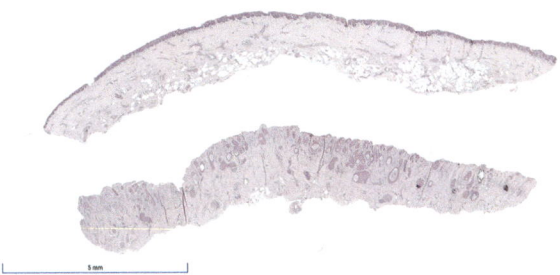

Fig. 33.4 Keratin-filled
cysts in the dermis,
mid-power

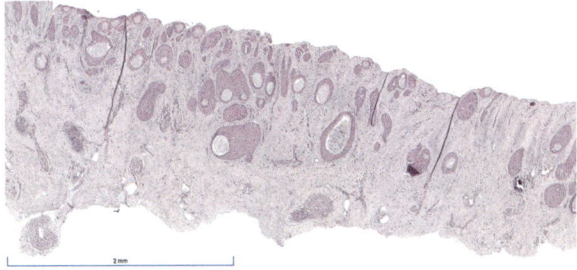

Fig. 33.5 Keratin-filled cysts lined with squamous epithelium, high-power

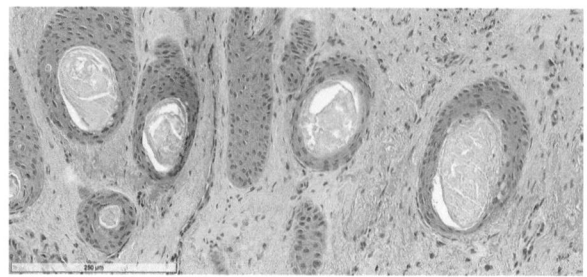

Based on the Case Description and the Photographs, What Is Your Diagnosis?

Melanoma
Pigmented Squamous Cell Carcinoma
Subungual Onycholemmal Cyst
Nevus
Lentigo
Subungual Fibrous Histiocytoma
Onychomycosis

Diagnosis

Subungual Onycholemmal Cyst

Discussion

Subungual onycholemmal cysts are also termed subungual epidermoid cysts or sub-ungual epidermoid inclusions [1]. This entity was first described in 1959 and it is a rare condition arising from the nail bed [2]. The clinical presentation is variable; it may manifest as nail-plate thickening and shortening, ridging, clubbing, subungual hyperkeratosis, onycholysis, or a pigmented band, as in our case [1, 3, 4]. In some patients, the nail appears normal and the onycholemmal cysts are only identified as an incidental finding on pathology. Although onycholemmal cysts are typically asymptomatic, they may also be painful. The great toenail or thumbnail are the most commonly affected nails. Many patients identify preceding trauma to the nail, although it is not clear if this is a causative factor [3].

Diagnosis is made through nail bed or nail matrix biopsy, which is often per-formed to rule out melanoma or other malignant nail tumors. Other differential diagnoses may include squamous cell carcinoma, nevus, lentigo, subungual fibrous histiocytoma, psoriasis, lichen planus, or onychomycosis.

On pathology, nail bed hyperkeratosis and acanthosis may be seen along with multiple small keratin-filled cysts in the dermis [2, 3]. These cysts typically lack a granular layer as they are derived from the nail bed epithelium, which also lacks a granular layer [4]. Calcification within the cysts has been reported [5]. Histologically, onycholemmal cysts must be distinguished from onycholemmal carcinomas which display atypical squamous epithelium lining the cysts along with nests of atypical keratinocytes within the dermis [4, 6].

Subungual onycholemmal cysts are benign and do not require further treatment. If the lesion is symptomatic, then the patient may opt for elective excision [7]. It is important to be aware of this nail abnormality as subungual onycholemmal cysts are likely underdiagnosed as their clinical appearance is variable and often mimics other conditions.

Key Points

- Subungual onycholemmal cysts are rare, benign nail bed growths that can present with a wide variety of clinical findings.
- This entity may present clinically as a pigmented band. In these cases, nail biopsy may be warranted to distinguish it from melanoma.
- Histologically, numerous small keratin-filled cysts can be seen in the dermis and may be accompanied by nail bed hyperkeratosis and acanthosis.

References

1. Lydrup E, Pederson Pilt A, Volker-Jürgen S, Trøstrup H. Subungual onycholemmal cysts: a case report. Case Rep Dermatol. 2021;13(2):394–8.
2. Samman PD. The human toe nail. Its genesis and blood supply. Br J Dermatol. 1959;71(8–9):296–302.
3. Fanti PA, Tosti A. Subungual epidermoid inclusions: report of 8 cases. Dermatologica. 1989;178:209–12.
4. Busquets J, Banala M, Campanelli C, Sahu J, Lee JB. Subungual onycholemmal cyst of the toenail mimicking subungual melanoma. Cutis. 2016;98(2):107–10.
5. Telang GH, Jellineck N. Multiple calcified subungual epidermoid inclusions. J Am Acad Dermatol. 2007;56(2):336–9.
6. Alessi E, Coggi A, Gianottie R, Parafioriti A, Berti E. Onycholemmal carcinoma. Am J Dermatopathol. 2004;26(5):397–402.
7. Sáez-de-Ocariz MM, Domínguez-Cherit J, García-Corona C. Subungual epidermoid cysts. Int J Dermatol. 2008;40(8):524–6.

Chapter 34
Nail Findings in an Expectant Mother

Marita Yaghi and Antonella Tosti

Abstract Fingernail onychomycosis can be difficult to diagnose as nail changes can closely resemble nail psoriasis. The disease can affect one or several nails and is usually limited to one hand. Toenail disease is often associate. Dermoscopy is helpful for diagnosis showing yellow patches.

Keywords Tinea unguium · Dermatophytes · Crumbling · Onycholysis · Onychoscopy

Clinical Case

A 26-year-old pregnant P2G3 female presented to the clinic with concerns about nail changes, initially noticed on her left thumb 4 years ago. The changes progressively involved the left-hand fingernails, sparing the fourth, and also affected all ten toenails. She had not been prescribed any treatment and denied using any over-the-counter product to treat her condition. The patient denied additional symptoms such as itch, skin rash, or joint pains, and her past medical history was unremarkable, except for two normal vaginal deliveries. She denied any history of known allergies and her only medications were prenatal vitamins.

Upon focused physical examination, all affected four left fingernails displayed thickening, yellowing, crumbling with partial destruction of the nail plate, leukonychia, and onycholysis. Dermoscopy (Handyscope 20 and 50X) examination of the fingernails showed partial destruction of the nail plate, yellow patches and white opaque discoloration of the nail plate and subungual scales. The plantar aspect of both feet showed fine scaling. Although the presence of nail polish limited the comprehensive assessment of toenail changes, nail plate thickening was evident. A

M. Yaghi · A. Tosti (✉)
Dr. Phillip Frost Department of Dermatology and Cutaneous Surgery, University of Miami Miller School of Medicine, Miami, FL, USA
e-mail: Mxy537@med.miami.edu; atosti@med.miami.edu

© The Author(s), under exclusive license to Springer Nature Switzerland AG 2025
A. Tosti et al. (eds.), *Clinical Cases in Nail Disorders*, Clinical Cases in Dermatology, https://doi.org/10.1007/978-3-031-88642-3_34

Fig. 34.1 Clinical photograph of the left-hand showing fingernail thickening, yellowing, crumbling, leukonychia, and onycholysis

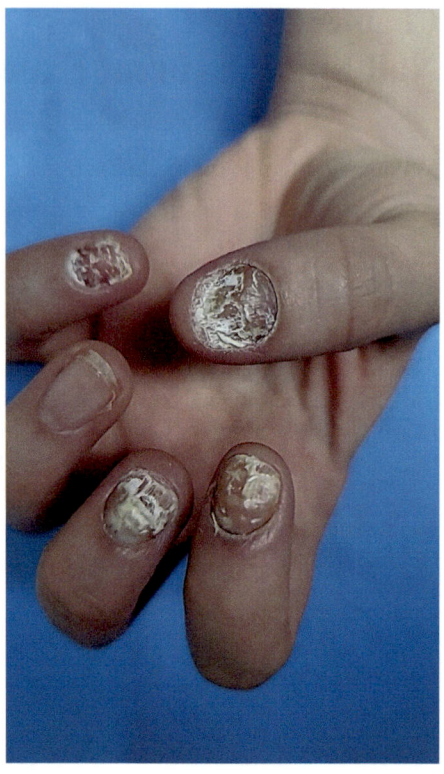

comprehensive full-body skin, hair, and nail examination revealed no additional abnormal findings.

Nail clippings obtained from both the left third fingernail and right great toenail were submitted for histopathological examination and fungal culture (Figs. 34.1, 34.2, 34.3, 34.4 and 34.5).

Based on the Case Description and the Photographs, What Is Your Diagnosis?

A. Nail psoriasis
B. Contact dermatitis secondary to acrylic nails
C. Twenty-nail dystrophy
D. Onychomycosis
E. Pregnancy-induced nail dystrophy

Fig. 34.2 Dermoscopy captures showing yellow patches, leukonychia, onycholysis and subungual scaling (20× magnification)

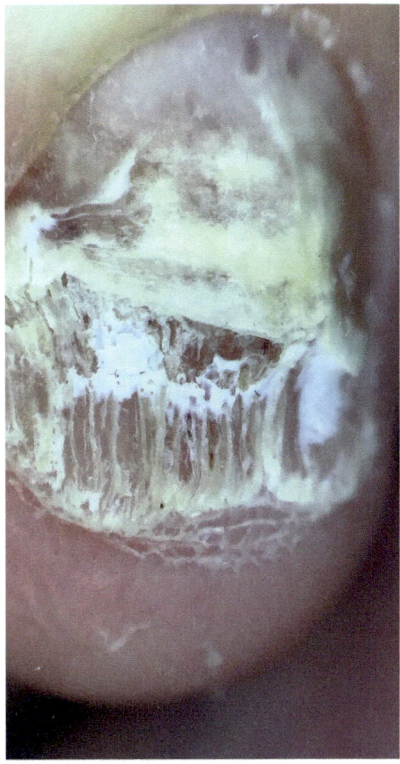

Diagnosis

Onychomycosis

Fungal culture identified the presence of Trichophyton rubrum in the collected specimen. Periodic acid-Schiff staining of nail fragments revealed the presence of numerous septate hyphae within the nail upon microscopic examination.

Discussion

Onychomycosis, constituting approximately 50% of nail diseases, exhibits a global prevalence of up to 10% [1, 2]. This persistent fungal infection primarily targets the toenails, with most common type being distal subungual onychomycosis (DSO) [3]. This type occurs when fungal invasion originates from the distal or lateral undersurface of the nail plate. Fingernail involvement is much less common and clinical features typically seen in DSO such as onycholysis with yellow streaks and subungual hyperkeratosis are not usually evident, making the differential diagnosis with

Fig. 34.3 Dermoscopy
captures showing almost
complete absence of the
nail plate due to
onycholysys and nail bed
scaling (20× magnification)

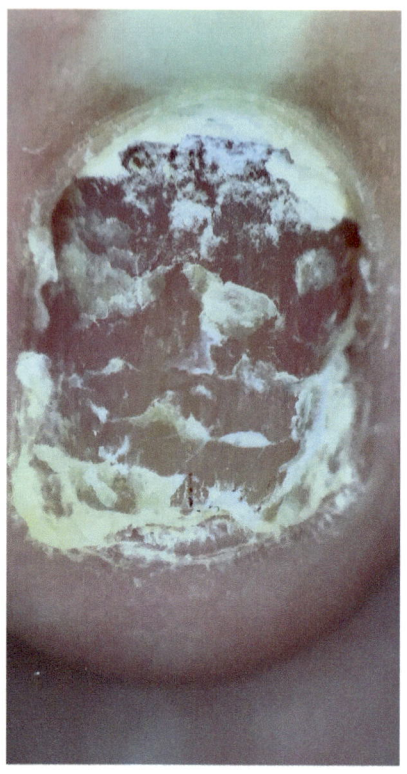

other nail disorders much more difficult. Presence of yellow patches at dermoscopy suggested the diagnosis in this case. It is important to keep in mind that is very typical for fingernail onychomycosis to affect fingernail of a single hand togheter with toenails of both feet "one hand and two feet syndrome". Scaling of the plantar areas is also characteristic. This case underlines the clinical difficulties in recognizing fingernail onychomycosis that can easily be misdiagnosed with many other nail conditions, particularly psoriasis and the importance of perform fungal stains and culture in nail changes limited to one hand.

The visualization of numerous septate hyphae within the nail plate, observed through Periodic acid-Schiff (PAS) stain, provides clear evidence of fungal involvement.

Fingernails tend to respond well to treatment with oral antifungals with mycological cure rates reaching up to 79% and complete cure rates ranging from 47% to 59% [4].

An important consideration is the association of these oral antifungals with congenital abnormalities in the fetus and spontaneous abortions, warranting against their use during pregnancy [5]. Additionally, both terbinafine and itraconazole harbor a concern of accumulation with nursing infants at high doses when used postpartum during breastfeeding [6].

Fig. 34.4 Dermoscopy
captures showing absence
of the nail plate and nail
bed scaling (20×
magnification)

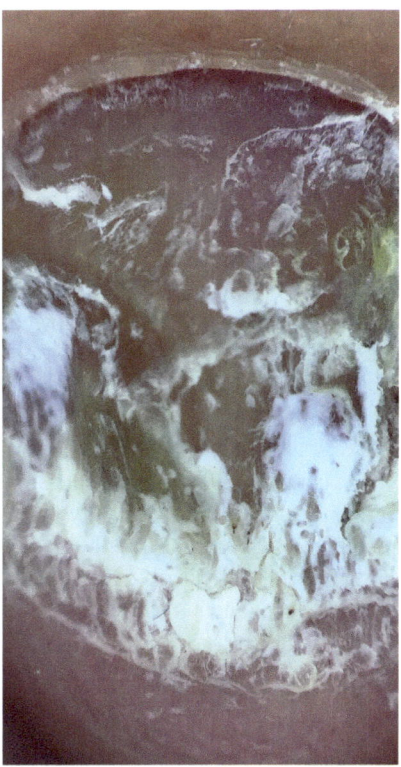

Key Points

- Fingernail onychomycosis, though less frequent than toenail involvement, still presents a significant clinical burden globally, affecting a notable proportion of the population.
- Fingernail onychomycosis typically manifests with symptoms such as yellowish discoloration, nail plate destruction, and onycholysis, which may impact the aesthetic appearance and functionality of the affected nails.
- Distinguishing fingernail onychomycosis from other nail conditions like ungual psoriasis can be challenging due to overlapping clinical features, but careful examination and laboratory tests such as fungal culture or histopathology are essential for accurate diagnosis.
- Fingernail onychomycosis requires oral antifungal therapy with terbinafine oritraconazole for effective eradication, and treatment tends to achieve higher mycologic and cure rates in fingernails compared to toenails.
- Emerging resistance to oral antifungals emphasizes the need for alternative treatments like topical efinaconazole, which has demonstrated superior efficacy in clinical trials, offering hope for improved outcomes in onychomycosis management.

Fig. 34.5 Dermoscopy captures showing yellow patches (20× magnification)

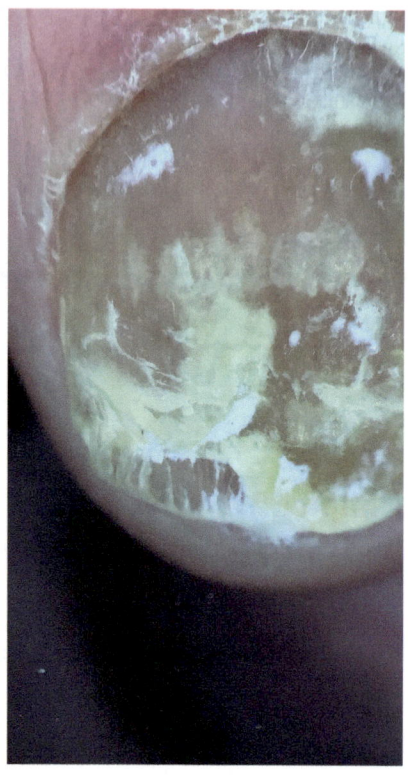

References

1. Sigurgeirsson B, Baran R. The prevalence of onychomycosis in the global population–a literature study. J Eur Acad Dermatol Venereol. 2014;28(11):1480–91.
2. Thomas J, Jacobson G, Narkowicz C, Peterson G, Burnet H, Sharpe C. Toenail onychomycosis: an important global disease burden. J Clin Pharm Ther. 2010;35(5):497–519.
3. Maskan Bermudez N, Rodríguez-Tamez G, Perez S, Tosti A. Onychomycosis: old and new. J Fungi. 2023;9(5):559.
4. Lipner SR, Scher RK. Onychomycosis: treatment and prevention of recurrence. J Am Acad Dermatol. 2019;80(4):853–67.
5. McMullan P, Yaghi M, Truong TM, Rothe M, Murase J, Grant-Kels JM. Safety of dermatologic medications in pregnancy and lactation: an update-Part I: pregnancy. J Am Acad Dermatol. 2024;
6. Yaghi M, McMullan P, Truong TM, Rothe M, Murase J, Grant-Kels JM. Safety of dermatologic medications in pregnancy and lactation: An Update-Part II: Lactation. J Am Acad Dermatol. 2024;91:651.

Chapter 35
Longitudinal Melanonychia of Left Hand Thumb Nail After Contact Dermatitis

Gamze Togac (iD), Fatih Ay (iD), and Umit Tursen (iD)

Abstract Melanonychia is pigmentation of the nail plate due to melanocyte activation or proliferation. Longitudinal melanonychia is the most common pattern. There are many etiologic factors depending on the number of nails involved and the dermoscopic features of the nail. These include trauma, infection, malignancy, pregnancy, dermatologic diseases, and medications (Jefferson J, Rich P. PMID: 22792094, PMCID: PMC3390039. In: Melanonychia. https://doi.org/10.1155/2012/952186). One or more than one fingernails or toenails may be involved and may occur at any age.

The history and clinical and dermoscopic features are instructive as to whether it is benign or malignant (Baykal C. Atlas of dermatology. 4th ed).

Melanonychia may present as a longitudinal band, transverse band or total melanonychia involving the entire nail. Since melanonychia requires biopsy for definitive diagnosis and biopsy can be invasive and may lead to nail dystrophies, biopsy is not performed in all lesions. Clinical examination and dermoscopic findings help to make the correct diagnosis and reduce the number of unnecessary surgeries (Demirdağ HG, Akay BN. Melanonychia. In: Türkiye Klinikleri, pp 16–22, 2020).

Melanocytes are found in the matrix and nail bed. The majority of these melanocytes are inactive. When triggered by trauma, infection, inflammation, etc., melanocytes are activated, begin to synthesize melanin and these melanin-rich melanosomes are transferred along dendrites to matrix cells. These matrix cells move distally and appear as pigmentation in the nail bed. Melanocytes also proliferate to form structures such as nevi, lentigo and malignant melanoma (Jefferson J, Rich P. PMID: 22792094, PMCID: PMC3390039. In: Melanonychia. https://doi.org/10.1155/2012/952186).

Discussion

Our patient with homogeneous regular longitudinal melanonychia on the first nail of the left hand was treated for contact dermatitis, the lesion was recorded on the dermoscopy device and she was called for follow-up after 3 months. As in our case, melanonychia may be triggered by contact dermatitis followed by nail find-

G. Togac · F. Ay · U. Tursen (✉)
Department of Dermatology, Mersin University, Mersin, Turkey

A. Tosti et al. (eds.), *Clinical Cases in Nail Disorders*, Clinical Cases in Dermatology, https://doi.org/10.1007/978-3-031-88642-3_35

ings. Trauma, various infections, pregnancy, drug exposure, malignant causes may play a role in the etiology of melanonychia.

Keywords Contact dermatitis · Melanonychia · Malignant melanoma

Clinical Case

A 66-year-old woman presented with a complaint of nail discoloration on the 1st nail plate of the left hand for 2 months. There was no history of trauma. The patient told that the lesion did not change color and did not grow. There was longitudinal hyperpigmentation on the nail plate and he had contact dermatitis and nail breakage, clefting, beau lines and chronic paronychia in the hand for 5 months (Fig. 35.1). Huntchinson's sign was negative. There was no history of trauma. There was no drug history. Hyphae examination of the nail was negative. The patient was not receiving any treatment for contact dermatitis and had intense chemical exposure such as detergents. Nail dermoscopy revealed homogeneous colored longitudinal regular bands on the first nail of the left hand (Fig. 35.2). There was no pigmentation in the other nails. Ferritin and B12 levels were normal.

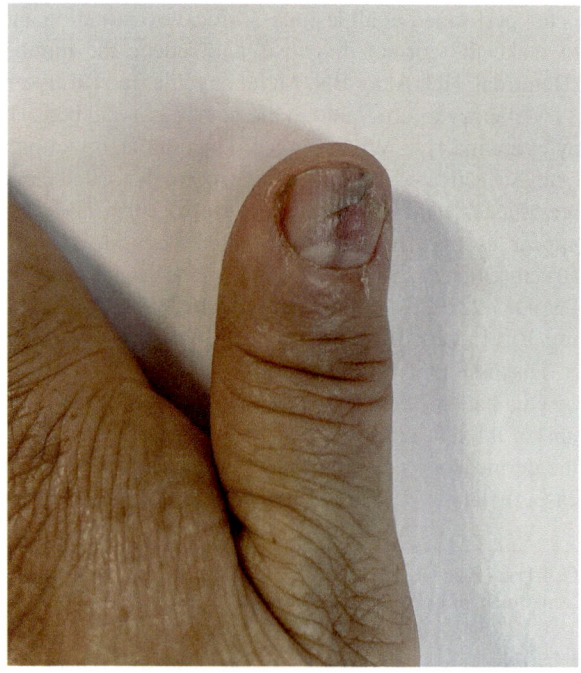

Fig. 35.1 Longitudinal hyperpigmentation and nail changes in the first nail of the left hand

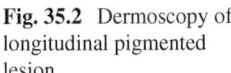

Fig. 35.2 Dermoscopy of longitudinal pigmented lesion

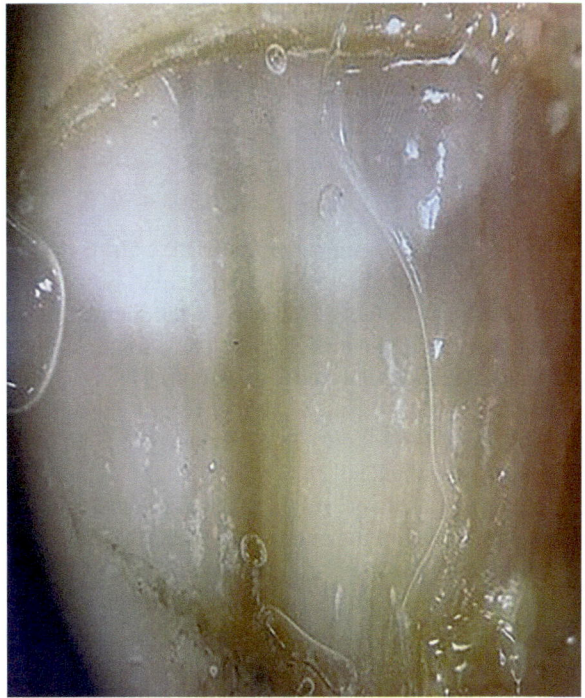

Based on the Case Description and the Photographs, What Is Your Diagnosis?

1. Longitudinal Melanonychia of left hand thumb nail after contact dermatitis
2. Subungal Melanoma
3. Subungal Hematoma

Diagnosis

Longitudinal Melanonychia of left hand thumb nail after contact dermatitis

Discussion

Our patient with homogeneous regular longitudinal melanonychia on the first nail of the left hand was treated for contact dermatitis, the lesion was recorded on the dermoscopy device and she was called for follow-up after 3 months. As in our case, melanonychia may be triggered by contact dermatitis followed by nail findings.

Table 35.1 Table of contact dermatitis nail findings

Subungal hyperkeratosis (common)
Onycholysis (common)
Chronic paronychia
Beau lines
Pitting
Melanonychia (rarely)

Melanonychia is pigmentation of the nail plate due to melanocyte activation or proliferation. Longitudinal melanonychia is the most common pattern. There are many etiologic factors depending on the number of nails involved and the dermoscopic features of the nail. These include trauma, infection, malignancy, pregnancy, dermatologic diseases, and medications [1]. One or more than one fingernails or toenails may be involved and may occur at any age.

The history and clinical and dermoscopic features are instructive as to whether it is benign or malignant [2].

Melanonychia may present as a longitudinal band, transverse band or total melanonychia involving the entire nail. Since melanonychia requires biopsy for definitive diagnosis and biopsy can be invasive and may lead to nail dystrophies, biopsy is not performed in all lesions. Clinical examination and dermoscopic findings help to make the correct diagnosis and reduce the number of unnecessary surgeries [3].

Melanocytes are found in the matrix and nail bed. The majority of these melanocytes are inactive. When triggered by trauma, infection, inflammation, etc., melanocytes are activated, begin to synthesize melanin and these melanin-rich melanosomes are transferred along dendrites to matrix cells. These matrix cells move distally and appear as pigmentation in the nail bed. Melanocytes also proliferate to form structures such as nevi, lentigo and malignant melanoma [1]. Trauma, various infections, pregnancy, drug exposure, malignant causes may play a role in the etiology of melanonychia.

One of the etiological causes that triggers melanonychia is contact dermatitis. Although it is known that contact dermatitis can cause onycholysis, subungual hyperkeratosis, pitting and beau lines in the nail, it can rarely cause melanonychia (Table 35.1). Understanding the potential triggers and mechanisms underlying melanonychia development is essential for accurate diagnosis and management of nail disorders.

Key Points

This case highlights the potential association between longitudinal melanonychia and contact dermatitis. The patient's history of intense chemical exposure and the presence of nail breakage, clefting, beau lines, and chronic paronychia suggest a link between the two conditions.

The absence of Hutchinson's sign, negative hyphae examination, normal ferritin and B12 levels, and the patient's lack of history of trauma or drug use helped exclude underlying malignancy. This underscores the importance of thorough clinical evaluation to differentiate benign from malignant causes of melanonychia.

Treating the underlying contact dermatitis was a key aspect of managing this case. By addressing the trigger factor, the progression of nail findings associated with melanonychia may be halted or minimized.

Regular follow-up is essential in cases of melanonychia to monitor any changes in nail pigmentation and overall condition. This ensures timely intervention and management of any underlying conditions or complications that may arise.

References

1. Jefferson J, Rich P. PMID: 22792094, PMCID: PMC3390039. In: Melanonychia. https://doi.org/10.1155/2012/952186.
2. Baykal C. Atlas of dermatology. 4th ed.
3. Demirdağ HG, Akay BN. Melanonychia. In: Türkiye Klinikleri; 2020. p. 16–22.

Chapter 36
Onychomadesis of Multiple Nails Secondary to Quinolone

Ayse Nur Saribas Yildirim ⓘ **and Umit Tursen** ⓘ

Abstract An 81 years old man with known temporal arteritis who has been taking azothiopurine was admitted to our clinic with the complaint of changes in his fingernails. He was treated with intravenous levofloxacin for pneumonia 2 months before the nail change. A skin rash developed on the 5th day of treatment and resolved spontaneously in 1 week. Two months later, nail deformity started to develop. Dermatologic examination revealed onychomadesis, beau lines, yellow discoloration, subungual hyperkeratosis and erythema in the perineum of the nails of the hands and feet.

Discussion

Many drug classes have been associated with drug-induced nail abnormalities. Onychomadesis describes the presence of a transverse whole-thickness sulcus that divides the nail into 2 parts. Onychomadesis represents the extreme degree of Beau's lines and shares the same pathogenesis, which a temporary arrest of nail matrix mitotic activity. Local trauma to the nail bed is the most common cause of single-digit onychomadesis. In our case, there was no systemic or dermatologic disease in the etiology of onychomadesis. Onychomadesis developing after quinolone group antibiotherapy was diagnosed with the patient's medical history and dermatologic examination. Drug-induced nail abnormalities are usually transitory and disappear with drug withdrawal, but sometimes persist in time.

Keywords Onychomadesis · Drug eruption · Quinolone · Nail abnormalities

A. N. S. Yildirim · U. Tursen (✉)
Department of Dermatology, Mersin University, Mersin, Turkey

© The Author(s), under exclusive license to Springer Nature Switzerland AG 2025
A. Tosti et al. (eds.), *Clinical Cases in Nail Disorders*, Clinical Cases in Dermatology, https://doi.org/10.1007/978-3-031-88642-3_36

An 81 years old man with known temporal arteritis who has been taking azo-thiopurine was admitted to our clinic with the complaint of changes in his fin-gernails. It was learned that he had a localized rash on the trunk on two separate occasions and nail deformity occurred 2 months after the rash. He was treated with intravenous levofloxacin for pneumonia 2 months before the nail change. A skin rash developed on the 5th day of treatment and resolved spontaneously in 1 week. Two months later, nail deformity started to develop. After the second time pulmonary infection, which recurred 4 months after the first infection, he was treated with moxifloxacin from the quinalone group again. The complaint of localized rash on the trunk recurred and nail changes continued. Dermatologic examination revealed onychomadesis, beau lines, yellow discoloration, subungual hyperkeratosis and erythema in the perineum of the nails of the hands and feet. (Figs. 36.1, 36.2 and 36.3) No fungal elements were found in the native preparation of the fingernails and toenails. There were 2 separate beau lines on the dermoscopic image of hand nail plate indicating 2 different periods. (Fig. 36.4).

Fig. 36.1 Onychomadesis of the entire fingernails

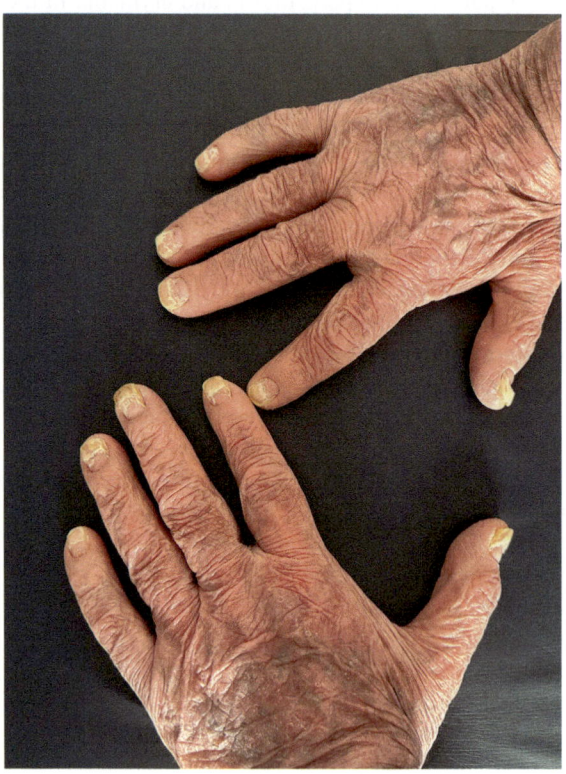

Fig. 36.2 The beau line seen on the fingernails, two pieces parallel to each other

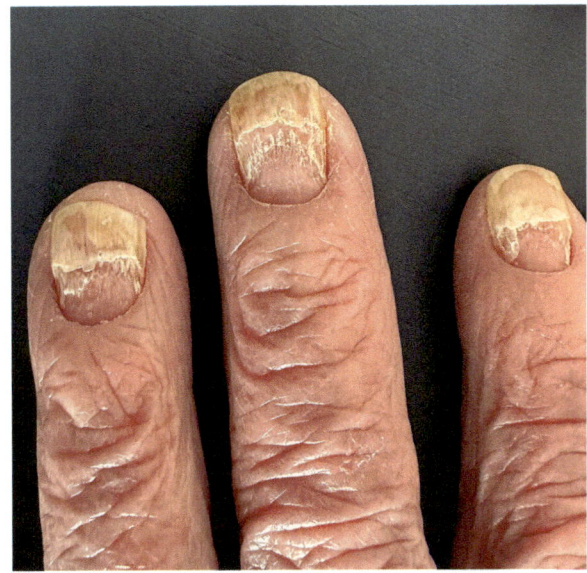

Fig. 36.3 Onychomadesis of toenails

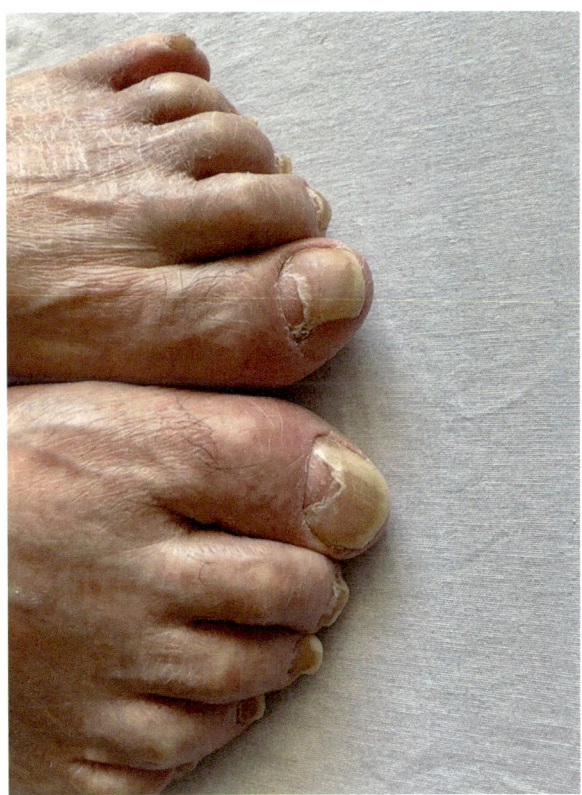

Fig. 36.4 Dermoscopic image

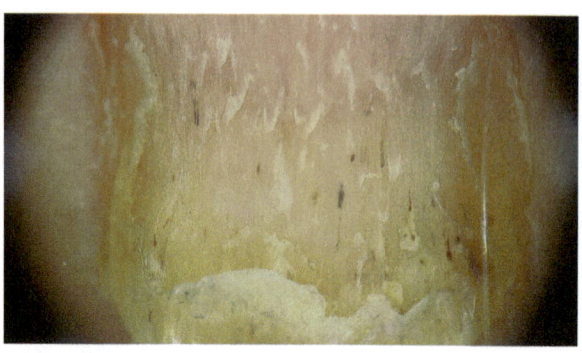

Based on the Case Description and the Photography, What Is Your Diagnosis?

1. Drug-induced oncyhomadesis
2. Twenty nail dystrophy
3. Onychomycosis

Diagnosis

1. Drug-induced oncyhomadesis

Discussion

Many drug classes have been associated with drug-induced nail abnormalities, including antimicrobials, antimalarials, cardiovascular agents, anti-inflammatories, antirheumatics, hormones, neuropsychiatric medications, as well as other agents. The specific nail dystrophic changes that result with each individual agent is determined by the portion of the nail apparatus affected. Photonycholysis, chromonychia, dyspigmentation of the nail unit, altered growth rate, Beaus' lines, onychomadesis, paronychia, and periungual pyogenic granulomas represent many common nail changes associated with systemic therapy [1]. Onychomadesis describes the presence of a transverse whole-thickness sulcus that divides the nail into 2 parts. Onychomadesis represents the extreme degree of Beau's lines and shares the same pathogenesis, which a temporary arrest of nail matrix mitotic activity. Local trauma to the nail bed is the most common cause of single-digit onychomadesis [2].

Table 36.1 Causes of onychomadesis

Etiology	Possible causes
Infectious	Hand-foot-and-mouth disease, varicella infection, scarlet fever, fungal infections
Systemic/ dermatologic	Periungual dermatitis, Stevens-Johnson syndrome, toxic epidermal necrolysis, lichen planus, Kawasaki disease
Drug related	Chemotherapeutic agents, valproic acid, carbamazepine, lithium, azithromycin
Other	Nail trauma, familial causes, idiopathic causes

Multiple-digit involvement suggests a systemic etiology such as fever, erythroderma, and Kawasaki disease; use of drugs (eg, chemotherapeutic agents, anticonvul¬sants, lithium, retinoids); and viral infections such as HFMD and varicella at the infantile age. Systemic and dermatological diseases such as periungual dermatitis, Stevens-Johnson syndrome, toxic epidermal necrolysis, lichen planus, Kawasaki disease may also cause onychomadesis [2] (Table 36.1).

All drugs responsible for the development of Beau's lines may cause the appearance of ony chomadesis, depending on the dosage of the drug and possibly on the patients' conditions [3].

In our case, there was no systemic or dermatologic disease in the etiology of onychomadesis. The patient did not describe a history of trauma, chemotherapy treatment or viral infection. Only levofloxacin and moxifloxacin treatments administered in 2 different periods were available. Onychomadesis developing after quinolone group antibiotherapy was diagnosed with the patient's medical history and dermatologic examination. The patient was told that the nail deformity would regress over time and might relapse after quinolone group antibiotherapy.

Drug-induced nail changes usually involve several or all 20 nails and appear in temporal correlation with drug intake. Drug-induced nail abnormalities are usually transitory and disappear with drug withdrawal, but sometimes persist in time [3]. There is no treatment for onychomadesis, which will gradually progress distally with the nail growth [3].

Key Points

- Onychomadesis can occur after skin diseases such as pemphigus vulgaris, alopecia areata, epidermolysis bullosa, viral infections such as hand foot and mouth disease, trauma, radiotherapy treatment and various drug treatments, especially chemotherapy drugs.
- Diagnosis is based on clinical presentation.
- It regresses spontaneously without scarring and does not require any treatment.

References

1. Yost JM. Nail reactions to antibiotics, antimalarials, and other medications. In: Rubin AI, Jellinek NJ, Daniel CR, Scher RK, editors. Scher and Daniel's nails. Cham: Springer; 2018. https://doi.org/10.1007/978-3-319-65649-6_28.
2. Salgado F, Handler MZ, Schwartz RA. Shedding light on onychomadesis. Cutis. 2017;99(1):33–6.
3. Piraccini BM, Tosti A. Drug-induced nail disorders: incidence, management and prognosis. Drug Saf. 1999;21(3):187–201. https://doi.org/10.2165/00002018-199921030-00004.

Chapter 37
Reddish-Brown Distal Band in Toenails-A Sign of Systemic Diseases

Tubanur Çetinarslan (ⒾD), Aylin Türel Ermertcan (ⒾD), and Umit Tursen (ⒾD)

Abstract Nail color changes may occur as a result of chronic diseases, infections, malignancies or drug use. Half-and-half nails that present clinically with proximal white zone and distal brownish sharp demarcation that parallel to the distal or free margin of the nail, could be associated with mostly chronic renal disease, as well as Kawasaki disease, hepatic cirrhosis, Crohn's disease, zinc deficiency and systemic chemotherapeutics. However, the pathogenesis of this nail finding is not clear. Herein we present a 58 year-old female patient with reddish-brown bands on the distal part of toenails.

Keywords Chronic renal failure · Half-and-half nails · Nail discoloration

58 year-old female patient referred to our Dermatology department due to nail discoloration for 3 years. On dermatological examination; there were reddish-brown bands on the distal part of toenails (Fig. 37.1). There was no history of trauma. There was no known diagnosis of malignancy and no history of chemotherapy treatment. She had a diagnosis of chronic kidney failure associated with diabetes mellitus and the patient was under hemodialysis treatment. On laboratory examination; blood urea was 154 mg/dL and serum creatinine was 6.7 mg/dL. Liver enzymes and blood lipids were mildly elevated: aspartate aminotransferase (AST) 62 IU/ L (normal 15–60) and alanine aminotransferase (ALT) 44 IU/L (normal 13–40), lactate dehydrogenase (LDH) 302 U/L (normal 110–295), total cholesterol 263 mg/dl (normal 0–200), low density lipid cholesterol (LDL) 165 mg/dl (normal 0–130),

T. Çetinarslan (✉) · A. T. Ermertcan
Department of Dermatology and Venereology, Manisa Celal Bayar University, Manisa, Turkey

U. Tursen
Department of Dermatology, Mersin University, Mersin, Turkey

© The Author(s), under exclusive license to Springer Nature Switzerland AG 2025
A. Tosti et al. (eds.), *Clinical Cases in Nail Disorders*, Clinical Cases in Dermatology, https://doi.org/10.1007/978-3-031-88642-3_37

Fig. 37.1 Reddish-brown bands on the distal part of toenails

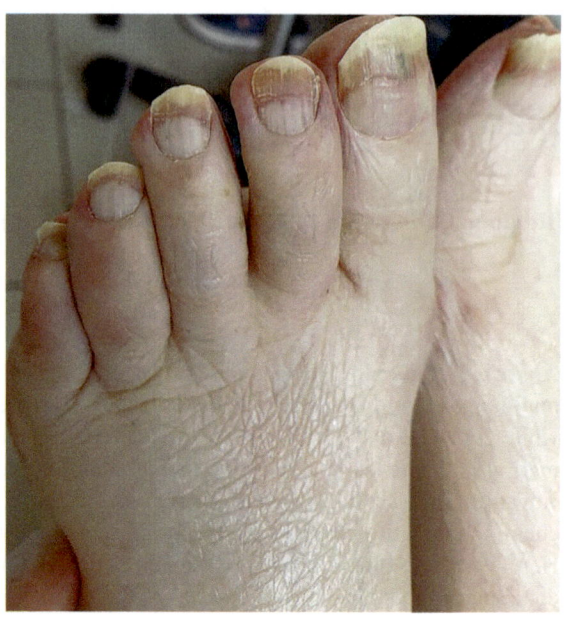

triglyceride 175 mg/dl (normal 0–150). There was no known family history of nail dystrophy or nail disease. The patient was being followed up in the Nephrology inpatient clinic and was consulted to the our Dermatology department for nail changes. What is your diagnosis?

Differential Diagnoses

1. Terry's Nails
2. Beau's lines
3. Yellow-nail syndrome
4. Half-and-half nails

Diagnosis

Half-and-half nails

Discussion

In 1967, Lindsay described half-and-half nails as a spsific clue of chronic kidney disease [1]. Half-and-half nails that present clinically with proximal white zone and distal brownish sharp demarcation that parallel to the distal or free margin of the nail, have been reported in 20–50% of patients with chronic renal disease [1, 2]. Half-and-half nails also have been reported in Kawasaki disease, hepatic cirrhosis, Crohn's disease, zinc deficiency, in patients treated with systemic chemotherapy [3–5], and as well as idiopathic form [6]. The pathogenesis of this nail finding is not clear [7]. It was suggested that this nail color change is caused by a nail bed pathology due to remained location of bands with nail growth [1]. Histopathologically, it is characterized by the increase of vessel wall thickness and melanin deposition in the distal half of the nail bed [1, 2, 7]. There is no relation between with severity of renal disease and occurance of half-and-half nails, as well as the length of the distal bands. Hemodialysis has no effect on half-and-half nails, however, it was reported to disappear completely within 3 weeks after kidney transplantation [8].

Key Points

In a patient with half-and-half nails, chronic renal failure should first be considered. Although this nail disorder only causes cosmetic problems, it is an important clue as it indicates underlying systemic diseases. A multidisciplinary approach is important in patients with half-and-half nails to detect underlying disorder.

References

1. Lindsay PG. The half-and-half nail. Arch Intern Med. 1967;119:583–7.
2. Stewart WK, Raffle EJ. Brown nail-bed arcs and chronic renal disease. Br Med J. 1972;1:784–6.
3. Pellegrino M, Taddeucci P, Mei S, Peccianti C. Half-and-half nail in apatient with Crohn's disease. J Eur Acad Dermatol Venereol. 2010;24:1366–7.
4. Afsar FS, Ozek G, Vergin C. Half-and-half nails in a pediatric patient after chemotherapy. Cutan Ocul Toxicol. 2015;34(4):350–1.
5. Iorizzo M, Daniel CR, Tosti A. Half and half nails: a past and present snapshot. Cutis. 2011;88:138–9.
6. Verma P, Mahajan G. Idiopathic 'Half and half' nails. J Eur Acad Dermatol Venereol. 2015 Jul;29(7):1452.
7. Das A, Choudhury S, Pandit S, Das SK. Medical image. Half-and-half nail. N Z Med J. 2012;125:103–4.
8. Leyden JJ, Wood MG. The "half-and-half nail" a uremic onychopathy. Arch Dermatol. 1972;105:591–2.

Chapter 38
Chronic Paronychia and Upward Growth of Nail Plates

Uwe Wollina 🔘

Abstract We report on a 28-year-old female with toenail problems. She suffered from chronic and painful paronychia. Her toenails were thickened and growing upwards in a 45 degree to the underlying bony phalanx. The nail disorder seemed to be provoked by indoor bouldering due to tight shoe fitting.

Keywords Chronic paronychia · Onychauxis · Upward positioning of the nail plate · Feet · Bouldering

Clinical Case

A 28-year-old woman presented in the outpatient clinic. She was concerned about her toenails which were growing upwards in a 45 degree to the underlying bony phalanx with chronic moderate painful inflammation since more than 12 months. Nail clipping was painful.

Her medical history was unremarkable. She had no regular medication, was of normosomeric physique and no trauma had been reported. As a leisure activity, she used to boulder, mainly indoor.

On examination, we observed an abnormal upward direction of nail's growth, most pronounced on digits III to V on both feet. This was accompanied by a chronic proximal fold (on some toes also on the medial and lateral nail fold)

U. Wollina (✉)
Department of Dermatology and Allergology, Städtisches Klinikum Dresden, Academic Teaching Hospital, Dresden, Germany

A. Tosti et al. (eds.), *Clinical Cases in Nail Disorders*, Clinical Cases in Dermatology, https://doi.org/10.1007/978-3-031-88642-3_38

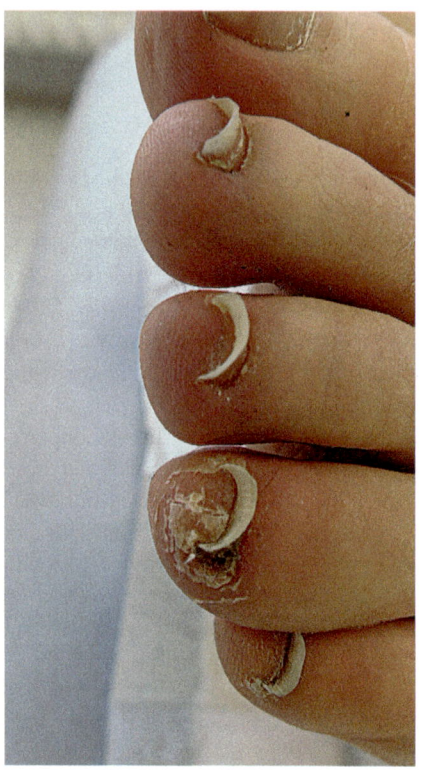

inflammation and presence of circumscribed hyperkeratosis of digits IV and V. The color of the nails plate was not changed. There were no signs of brittle nails. Both the cuticle and the hyponychium were missing on toes III to IV (Figs. 38.1, 38.2 and 38.3).

Fig. 38.1 Left foot with upwards growth of the nail plates and chronic nail fold inflammation. Hyperkeratotic bulbs on digit IV and V. Loss of cuticle on digit II to V

Fig. 38.2 Right foot. Upward growth of nail plates, chronic lateral and proximal paronychia. Loss of cuticle and hyponychium on digit III

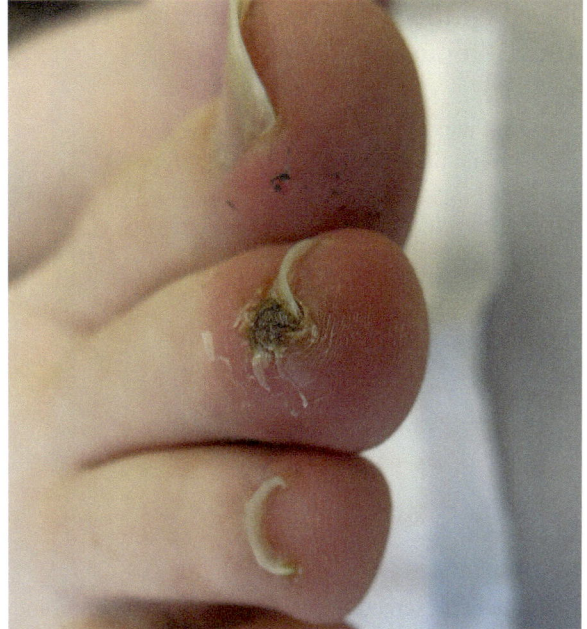

Fig. 38.3 Left Foot, digitus V. Double nail plate, upwards growth of the nail plate. Mild hyperkeratotic skin on the bulb. Loss of the hyponychium

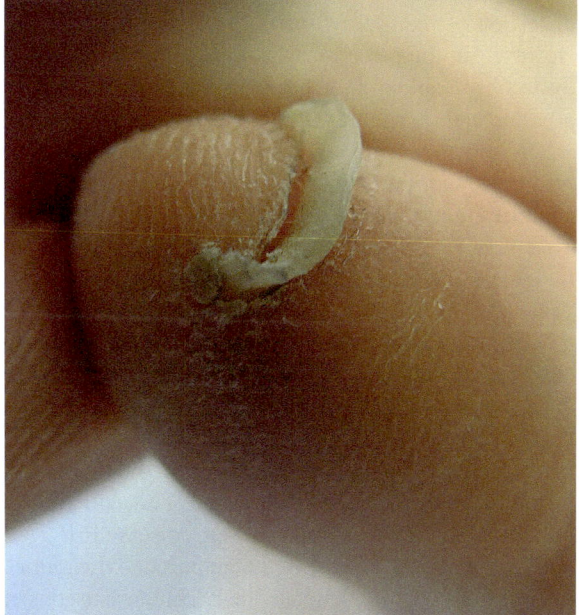

Based on the Case Description and the Photographs, What Is Your Diagnosis?

(a) Onychauxis
(b) Chronic paronychia with onychogryposis
(c) Distal onycholysis
(d) Koilonychia

Diagnosis

Chronic paronychia with onyogryposis.

Discussion

The patient presented a combination of painful chronic paronychia, nail plate thickening (onychauxis) and upward positioning of the nail plate on both feet. An abnormally short distal phalanx of the big toe in little children may lead to upward distortion of the nail as the pulp of the toe is dislodged dorsally during gait [1]. However, in the present case sports (bouldering) may have contributed to her nail dystrophy. Bouldering shoes are very tight. In predisposed people this may lead to pressure and friction resulting in repeated minor trauma.

Chronic paronychia (CP) is an inflammatory disorder of the nail folds persisting >6 weeks. Our patient achieved a CP score of 10 in the most affected toes [2]. In contrast to acute paronychia, CP is mostly non-suppurative and often multi-factorial. Treatment is difficult, even when one identified factor can be eliminated. Typical findings are loss of cuticle, variable degree of erythematous swelling, and pain [3]. Table 38.1 lists various etiologies and differential diagnoses.

The herein observed upwards positioning of toenails, however, is uncommon in CP. Mechanical factors of her sportive activity may have contributed. Some of her nails (Fig. 38.2) had a mild overcurvature suggesting an initial stage of pincer nail development. Pincer nails are thought to be due to a nailbed shrinkage [5]. This can be caused by mechanical forces. If nailbed shrinkage goes further proximal, the nail plate may lose contact to the nail bed. This will allow an upward positioning of the nail plate as seen in nail bed Bowen's disease [6].

We prescribed topical bethamethasone—fusidinic acid cream once a day for 6 weeks and recommended other leisure activities than bouldering, which was denied by the patient. There was a partial improvement—edema, erythema and pain were significantly reduced. The abnormal nail plate growth, however, cannot be corrected by conservative approaches if the distal nail bed is lost. In more initial

Table 38.1 Underlying disorders in CP [3, 4]

Diagnosis	Remarks
Occupational CP	Mostly seen in employees exposed to moisture and irritants
Immunosuppression	Various causes like diabetes mellitus, HIV/AIDS, rheumatic disorders, post-transplantation, during cancer therapies
Infections	Tuberculosis, leishmaniasis, HPV-warts, orf, candidosis, lues
Cancer	Squamous cell carcinoma, Bowen's disease, melanoma, metastasis
Vascular occlusive diseases	Winiwarter-Buerger disease, systemic scleroderma, peripheral artery disease
Skin diseases	Pemphigoid, psoriasis, chronic contact dermatitis, retronychia
Drug-related	Retinoids, EGF-receptor inhibitors, BRAF inhibitors, MEK inhibitors, VEGF inhibitors, mTOR inhibitors, anti-retroviral protease inhibitors, Bruton's kinase inhibitors
Leisure activities	Running, climbing, bouldering, hicking

stages double wires and other correcting devices are helpful. Nail surgery is possible, but an excellent outcome cannot be guaranteed [7]. Therefore, the patient rejected surgery.

Key Points

- CP is a multi-factorial inflammatory disease persistent >6 weeks.
- CP can lead to secondary nail plate changes.
- Onychogryposis can cause GP.
- Treatment consists of conservative and surgical options.

References

1. Haneke E. Toenails: where orthopedics and onychology meet. In: Baran RL, editor. Advances in nail disease and management. Updates in clinical dermatology. Cham: Springer; 2021. p. 71–85.
2. Atış G, Göktay F, Altan Ferhatoğlu Z, Kaynak E, Sevim Keçici A, Yaşar Ş, Aytekin S. A proposal for a new severity index for the evaluation of chronic paronychia. Skin Appendage Disord. 2018;5(1):32–7.
3. Relhan V, Bansal A. Acute and chronic paronychia revisited: a narrative review. J Cutan Aesthet Surg. 2022;15(1):1–16.
4. Wollina U. Systemic drug-induced chronic paronychia and periungual pyogenic granuloma. Indian Dermatol Online J. 2018;9(5):293–8.
5. Huang C, Huang R, Yu M, Guo W, Zhao Y, Li R, Zhu Z. Pincer nail deformity: clinical characteristics, causes, and managements. Biomed Res Int. 2020;2020:2939850.
6. Wollina U. Bowen's disease of the nail apparatus: a series of 8 patients and a literature review. Wien Med Wochenschr. 2015;165(19–20):401–5.
7. Pandhi D, Verma P. Nail avulsion: indications and methods (surgical nail avulsion). Indian J Dermatol Venereol Leprol. 2012;78(3):299–308.

Chapter 39
Scaling Skin with Vertical Nail Plate Growth

Uwe Wollina ⓘ

Abstract A 51-year-old male patient was referred from the stroke unit to dermatological examination because of skin and nail disease of the affected leg. The patient was as long-time smoker and had several risk factors for stroke. On examination we observed scaling on the affects foot and lower leg without erythema or pruritus. The great toe showed a vertical growth of a thickened, dystrophic nail plate. The nail bed was miniaturized. Because of gait problems associated with the stroke the diagnosis of an asymmetric gait nail unit syndrome (AGNUS) was confirmed. This is the result of asymmetric shoe pressure on the toes and foot caused by uneven flat feet that affect the gait. The pressure produces clinical changes in the toenails and can also affect the nail bed.

Keywords Stroke · Gait problems · Asymmetric gait nail unit syndrome · Dermatitis neglecta · Nail dystrophy

Clinical Case

A 51-year-old male patient was referred from the stroke unit to dermatological examination because of skin and nail disease of the affected leg. The patient had a long history of high arterial blood pressure, hyperlipidemia, and > 25 years of smoking. He suffered from venous thromboembolism.

U. Wollina (✉)
Department of Dermatology and Allergology, Städtisches Klinikum Dresden, Academic Teaching Hospital, Dresden, Germany

A. Tosti et al. (eds.), *Clinical Cases in Nail Disorders*, Clinical Cases in Dermatology, https://doi.org/10.1007/978-3-031-88642-3_39

On examination we observed a significant scaling on the affects foot and lower leg without erythema or pruritus (Fig. 39.1).

The great toe showed a vertical growth of a thickened, dystrophic nail plate. There were no signs of a chronic paronychia. The nail bed was miniaturized (Fig. 39.2).

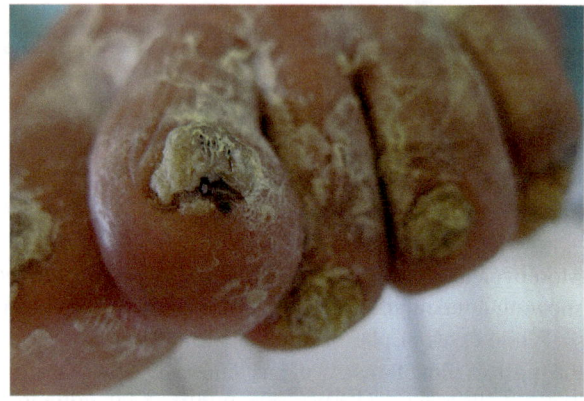

Fig. 39.1 Left foot. Dermatitis neglecta and great toenail dystrophy

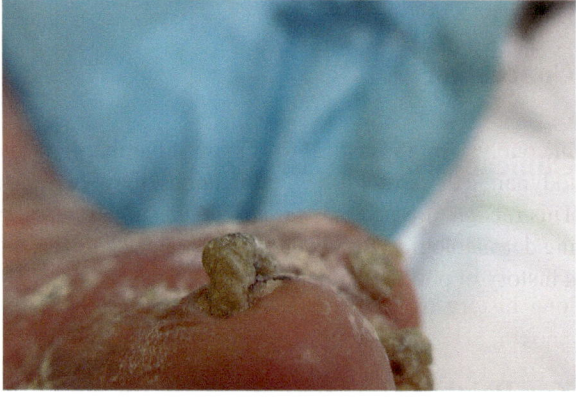

Fig. 39.2 Detail of the great toenail demonstrates a vertical growth of the nail plate

Based on the Case Description and the Photographs, What Is Your Diagnosis?

(a) Psoriasis
(b) Tinea pedum with onychomycosis
(c) Crusted scabies
(d) Onychodystrophy with dermatitis neglecta

Diagnosis

Onychodystrophy with dermatitis neglecta

Discussion

Stroke is a leading cause of long-term disability in the western world, with 50% of stroke survivors >65 years suffering from hemiparesis [1]. Patients with post-stroke hemiparesis exhibit impaired walking performance, characterized by slow walking speeds and asymmetrical spatiotemporal, kinematic, and kinetic patterns. Plantarflexor weakness is a common impairment in hemiparetic patients, changes gait biomechanics and limits gait speed [2].

Gait problems can cause secondary skin and nail changes [3, 4]. The most common example world-wide is the asymmetric gait nail unit syndrome (AGNUS) is the result of asymmetric shoe pressure on the toes and foot caused by uneven flat feet that affect the gait. The pressure produces clinical changes in the toenails, which are suggestive for onychomycosis, yet they are non-infectious [5]. Gait changes can also affect the nail bed. A nonfunctional nail bed loses the connection to the nail plate undersurface. Since the nail bed guides the growth direction of the nail plate, a loss of their tight interaction will allow the nail plate growing upwards. This has also been observed in malignant transformation of the nail bed in keratinocyte tumors [6].

Surgical nail avulsion would be an option for this condition if conservative measures are insufficient.

The scaling skin is the quite typical presentation of dermatitis neglecta, a benign dermatosis resulting from insufficient frictional cleansing of the skin. An accumulation of sebum, sweat, corneocytes, and residues of skin care products forming a compact and adherent crust on the skin surface [7]. Cleansing with soap water and improvement of personal hygiene are sufficient to treat this condition [8].

Key Points

- Micronychia can be a symptom of syndromic disease.
- Yellowish discolorations of the nail plate have many different causes.
- It is important to exclude the yellow nail syndrome.

References

1. Kelly-Hayes M, Beiser A, Kase CS, Scaramucci A, D'Agostino RB, Wolf PA. The influence of gender and age on disability following ischemic stroke: the Framingham study. J Stroke Cerebrovasc Dis. 2003;12(3):119–26.
2. Nadeau S, Gravel D, Arsenault AB, Bourbonnais D. Plantarflexor weakness as a limiting factor of gait speed in stroke subjects and the compensating role of hip flexors. Clin Biomech (Bristol, Avon). 1999;14(2):125–35.
3. Wollina U, Mohr F, Schier F. Unilateral hyperhidrosis, callosities, and nail dystrophy in a boy with tethered spinal cord syndrome. Pediatr Dermatol. 1998;15(6):486–7.
4. Wollina U, Bula P. Longitudinal 'half-and-half nails' or true leukonychia. Skin Appendage Disord. 2016;1(4):185–6.
5. Zaias N, Rebell G, Escovar S. Asymmetric gait nail unit syndrome: the most common worldwide toenail abnormality and onychomycosis. Skinmed. 2014;12(4):217–23.
6. Wollina U. Bowen's disease of the nail apparatus: a series of 8 patients and a literature review. Wien Med Wochenschr. 2015;165(19–20):401–5.
7. Poskitt L, Wayte J, Wojnarowska F, Wilkinson JD. 'Dermatitis neglecta': unwashed dermatosis. Br J Dermatol. 1995;132(5):827–9.
8. Ghosh SK, Sarkar S, Mondal S, Das S. Clinical profile of dermatitis neglecta with special emphasis on psychiatric comorbidities: a case series of 22 patients from Eastern India. Indian J Psychiatry. 2022;64(6):599–604.

Chapter 40
Onychomatricoma with Clinical and Ultrasonographic Correlation

Ximena Wortsman (ID)

Abstract An onychomatricoma case with clinical and ultrasonographic correlation is presented. This case teaches this ungual benign tumor's typical clinical and ultrasonographic signs and discusses the main differential diagnoses.

Keywords Onychomatricoma · Ultrasound · Nail · Dermatology · Ultrasonography

Clinical Case

Clinical Description

A 63-year-old female has shown a painless, yellowish appearance and progressive thickening with longitudinal lines in the nail of the right index finger for 1 year and a half (Figs. 40.1, 40.2, 40.3, 40.4, 40.5, 40.6 and 40.7).

X. Wortsman (✉)
Institute for Diagnostic Imaging and Research of the Skin and Soft Tissues, Santiago, Chile

Department of Dermatology, Faculty of Medicine, Universidad de Chile, Santiago, Chile

Department of Dermatology, School of Medicine, Pontificia Universidad Catolica de Chile, Santiago, Chile

Department of Dermatology and Cutaneous Surgery, Miller School of Medicine, Miami, USA

© The Author(s), under exclusive license to Springer Nature Switzerland AG 2025
A. Tosti et al. (eds.), *Clinical Cases in Nail Disorders*, Clinical Cases in Dermatology, https://doi.org/10.1007/978-3-031-88642-3_40

233

Fig. 40.1 Clinical image of the right index nail of a 63-year-old female patient. She noticed a painless, yellowish color, thickening, and longitudinal lines that had grown progressively for 1.5 years

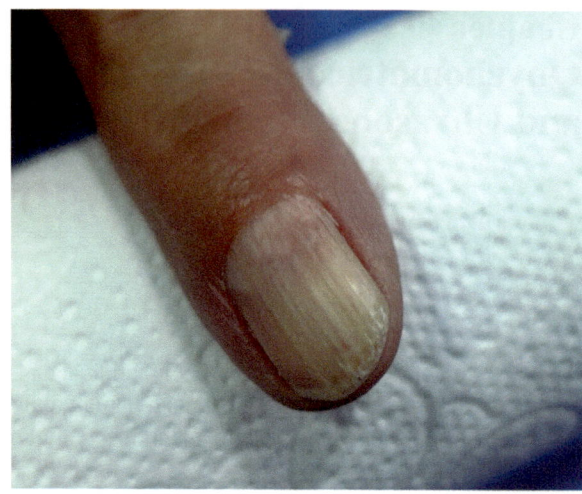

Fig. 40.2 Dermoscopy. Besides the previously commented findings, the dermoscopic view demonstrates erythema and some splinter hemorrhages

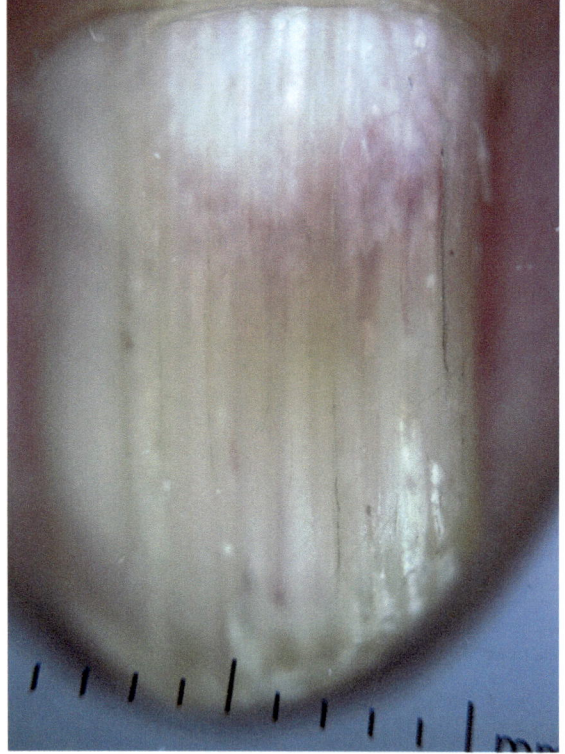

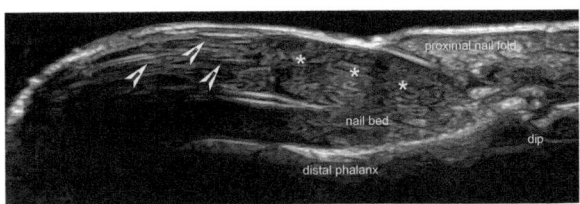

Fig. 40.3 Ultrasound at 24 MHz (greyscale, longitudinal view) shows an ill-defined hypoechoic mass (*) that protrudes into the nail plate and presents hyperechoic lines (arrows). A subtle scalloping of the bony margin of the distal phalanx is also detected without erosion of the bone. This ultrasound morphology is pathognomonic of onychomatricoma. The dimensions of the tumor were 1.5 cm (longitudinal) × 0.4 cm (thickness) × 0.9 cm (transverse). Abbreviation: dip, distal interphalangeal joint

Fig. 40.4 Ultrasound at 24 MHz (greyscale, transverse view) presents hyperechoic spots at the tumor site, corresponding to the hyperechoic lines detected in the longitudinal view

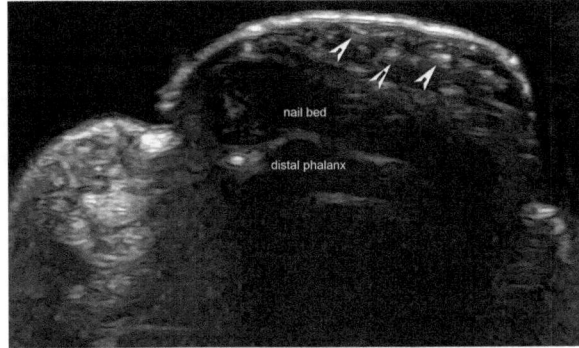

Fig. 40.5 Ultrasound at 70 MHz (greyscale; longitudinal view) zooms in on the subungual mass (*). Arrowheads mark some of the hyperechoic lines in the distal part of the tumor

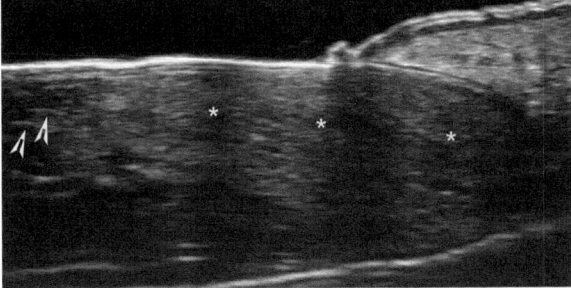

Fig. 40.6 Color Doppler ultrasound at 24 MHz (longitudinal view) shows a low degree of vascularity (colors) with the mass

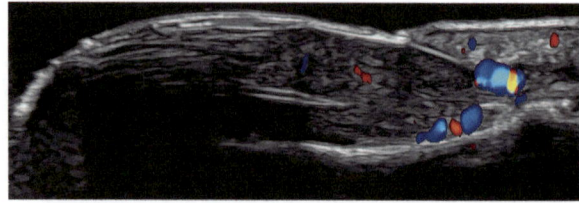

Fig. 40.7 Three-dimensional reconstruction (greyscale, longitudinal view) of the subungual mass (*). Notice the hyperechoic lines in the distal part of the lesion (arrows)

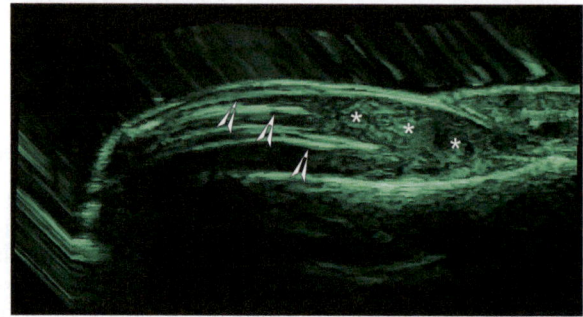

Color Doppler Ultrasound Report

A hypoechoic solid mass in the nail bed involves the matrix region and presents hyperechoic lines that protrude into the interplate space.

The mass measures 1.5 cm (longitudinal) × '0.4 cm (thickness) × 0.9 cm (transverse view).

Few vessels are observed within the mass, varying in thickness between 0.2 and 0.6 mm. They showed low-velocity arterial flow with a maximum peak systolic velocity of 4.8 cm/s.

The bony margin of the distal phalanx, the distal insertion of the extensor tendon, and the distal interphalangeal joint were unremarkable.

Ultrasound impression: These findings are compatible with an onychomatricoma.

Diagnosis

Onychomatricoma is a benign fibroepithelial tumor derived from the nail matrix that tends to affect middle-aged individuals. It is clinically characterized by slow-growing and painless xantonychia (yellowish color), longitudinal lines, proximal or distal splinter hemorrhages, overcurvature, and distal holes in the nail plate. [1–4]

Its clinical diagnosis may be challenging, particularly in early stages or pigmented variants [1, 2, 4].

On ultrasound, the reported onychomatricoma pattern was described in 2009 [5] and is composed of a hypoechoic hypovascular and usually eccentric mass that involves the matrix region, protrudes into the nail plate and presents hyperechoic lines (longitudinal) or spots (transverse). [5, 6] The pigmented variants of onychomatricoma are reported to present a similar ultrasonographic appearance [7].

The hyperechoic lines that penetrate into the nail plate correspond with the interphases of the finger-like projections of the tumor seen in surgery and pathology [5, 6].

The case presented was confirmed histopathologically.

Main Differential Diagnoses

The main differential clinical diagnoses include nail psoriasis, warts, and onychomycosis. However, they present different ultrasonographic patterns [6, 8].

Nail psoriasis shows a wide range of ultrasound morphologies according to the disease's degree of severity and activity. Among the ultrasound signs are the thickening of the nail bed, loss of definition of the ventral plate, irregularities, thickening and undulation of the nail plate. On color Doppler, a variable degree of hypervascularity is linked to the disease's inflammatory activity level. Additional findings can include anechoic fluid distention of the distal or proximal interphalangeal joints and the metacarpophalangeal joints (synovitis), hypoechogenicity of the insertion of the distal extensor tendon (enthesopathy), and erosions of the bony margin, which compose what is called psoriatic arthropathy [6, 9, 10].

The subungual nail warts usually present as a fusiform, eccentric, ill-defined, hypoechoic structure in the nail bed or periungual regions with upward displacement, thickening, and nail plate irregularities. No hyperechoic lines or spots are detected in the nail plate space; however, thickening and irregularities in the nail plate could be detected. According to the degree of severity of the disease, variable degrees of hypervascularity can be detected in the nail bed. This fusiform hypoechoic morphology is similar to that of warts that affect other corporal regions, such as the plantar region [6, 8, 9].

Onychomycosis can generate hypoechogenicity of the nail bed, but usually in the superficial part, as well as thickening and irregularities of the nail plate. In patients with concomitant onychomycosis and psoriasis, the nail beds tend to be thicker than onychomycosis and psoriasis alone. No erosions of the bony margin of the distal phalanx or synovitis have been reported on the ultrasound examinations of onychomycosis, which could also help to discriminate onychomycosis from psoriasis. On color Doppler, onychomycosis tends to be hypovascular [6, 9].

Key Points

- Ultrasound can support the diagnosis and extent of onychomatricoma in all axes.
- This includes the pigmented variants of onychomatricoma.
- The ultrasound pattern includes a hypoechoic hypovascular and usually eccentric mass that affects the nail matrix region and protrudes into the nail plate with hyperechoic lines or spots.

Conflict of Interest None.

Funding None.

References

1. Gam D, Jaka A, Ferrándiz C. Onychomatricoma: clinical, dermoscopy and ultrasound findings. Indian J Dermatol Venereol Leprol. 2019;85(2):190–1. https://doi.org/10.4103/ijdvl.IJDVL_621_17.
2. Schneider SL, Tosti A. Tips to diagnose uncommon nail disorders. Dermatol Clin. 2015;33(2):197–205. https://doi.org/10.1016/j.det.2014.12.003.
3. Starace M, Rubin AI, Di Chiacchio NG, et al. Diagnosis and surgical treatment of benign nail unit tumors. J Dtsch Dermatol Ges. 2023;21(2):116–29. https://doi.org/10.1111/ddg.14942.
4. Hare AQ, Rich P. Nail tumors. Dermatol Clin. 2021;39(2):281–92. https://doi.org/10.1016/j.det.2020.12.007.
5. Soto R, Wortsman X, Corredoira Y. Onychomatricoma: clinical and sonographic findings. Arch Dermatol. 2009;145(12):1461–2. https://doi.org/10.1001/archdermatol.2009.312.
6. Wortsman X. Concepts, role, and advances on nail imaging. Dermatol Clin. 2021;39(2):337–50. https://doi.org/10.1016/j.det.2020.12.010.
7. Peruilh-Bagolini L, Dossi MT, Wortsman X, Montero T. Pigmented onychomatricoma: a clinical simulator that could not mislead ultrasound. Acta Biomed. 2021;92(S1):e2021158. https://doi.org/10.23750/abm.v92iS1.9519.
8. Vargas EAT, Finato VML, Azulay-Abulafia L, Leverone A, Nakamura R, Wortsman X. Ultrasound of nails: why, how, when. Semin Ultrasound CT MR. 2023; https://doi.org/10.1053/j.sult.2023.11.004.
9. Wortsman X. Textbook of dermatologic ultrasound. 1st ed. Springer; 2022.
10. Agache M, Popescu CC, Enache L, Dumitrescu BM, Codreanu C. Nail ultrasound in psoriasis and psoriatic arthritis-a narrative review. Diagnostics (Basel). 2023;13(13) https://doi.org/10.3390/diagnostics13132236.

Chapter 41
Sarcoidosis of the Nail: The Greatest Imitator

Elizabeth Yim ⓘ**, Karen Lam** ⓘ**, and Gregory A. Gates** ⓘ

Abstract Nail involvement in sarcoidosis is rare, and usually observed in patients with systemic or cutaneous sarcoidosis. Treatment is often difficult with no clear guidelines and usually involves targeting systemic or cutaneous symptoms. In addition, nail sarcoidosis is often associated with underlying bony involvement and should warrant imaging in newly diagnosed patients. We present a case report of a 47-year-old male with a history of systemic sarcoidosis presenting with 1 year duration of nail dystrophy of his left big toenail. Biopsy of the nail revealed sarcoidosis of the nail. Interestingly, our patient did not have any osseous abnormalities of the underlying phalanx.

Keywords Sarcoidosis · Nail · Osseous · Granulomatous disease

E. Yim (✉)
Department of Internal Medicine, Division of Dermatology, University of Texas at Austin Dell Medical School, Austin, TX, USA
e-mail: Elizabeth.yim@austin.utexas.edu

K. Lam
Division of Dermatology, David Geffen School of Medicine, Los Angeles, CA, USA
e-mail: kalam@mednet.ucla.edu

G. A. Gates
Division of Dermatopathology, UCLA Medical Center, Department of Pathology and Laboratory Medicine, Los Angeles, CA, USA
e-mail: GAGates@mednet.ucla.edu

© The Author(s), under exclusive license to Springer Nature Switzerland AG 2025
A. Tosti et al. (eds.), *Clinical Cases in Nail Disorders*, Clinical Cases in Dermatology, https://doi.org/10.1007/978-3-031-88642-3_41

Clinical Case

A 47-year-old Caucasian male presented with painless discoloration and dystrophy of the left big toenail of one-year duration. His past medical history was significant for sarcoidosis diagnosed 13 years prior, when he developed bilateral uveitis, bilateral hilar and mediastinal lymphadenopathy, inguinal lymphadenopathy, and splenomegaly. A left femoral lymph node biopsy showed non-necrotizing epithelioid granulomas consistent with sarcoidosis. Cardiac magnetic resonance imaging (MRI) was negative for cardiac sarcoidosis. One year prior to presentation, the patient developed chronic pain and swelling of the right knee, and an MRI revealed sarcoid arthropathy of the right knee. Prior treatments included chronic prednisone 10 mg daily and tobramycin dexamethasone 0.3–0.1% eye drop treatments, resulting in remission of the patient's uveitis.

Physical exam demonstrated concavity of the toenail with longitudinal splitting, an erythematous proximal lunula, and a violaceous proximal nail fold (Fig. 41.1a, b). The differential diagnosis included lichen planus, sarcoidosis, amyloidosis, squamous cell carcinoma, and onychomycosis. A nail clipping was negative for bacterial and fungal organisms. Punch biopsy of the distal nail plate and nail bed was performed. Histopathology demonstrated ill-formed non-necrotizing granulomata with some "naked" granulomata which supported a diagnosis of sarcoidosis (Fig. 41.2a, b). X-ray of the left great toe revealed no bony abnormalities of the underlying distal phalanx. The patient was started on betamethasone dipropionate ointment 0.05% which he intermittently discontinued due to lack of improvement. Intralesional injection was offered but patient declined.

The patient also developed scaly, pink to slightly orange papules coalescing into annular plaques on the upper central forehead and left forehead and left cheek. A biopsy of one of these lesions showed granulomatous dermatitis which supported cutaneous sarcoidosis. Cutaneous sarcoidosis of the face was previously treated with liquid nitrogen and later 0.25 cc of intralesional triamcinolone 5 mg/mL into lesions on forehead and frontal scalp with no improvement noted by the patient but also no growth of further skin lesions. Patient reported cosmetic concerns due to these skin lesions but were otherwise asymptomatic.

Due to worsening sarcoid arthropathy of his right knee, the patient was transitioned to methotrexate 15 mg weekly with folic acid by his rheumatologist which led to improvement of his joint pain and continues at this dose. The patient was not able to tolerate a higher dose of methotrexate and patient deferred adding on hydroxychloroquine vs. adalimumab for better skin and nail improvement.

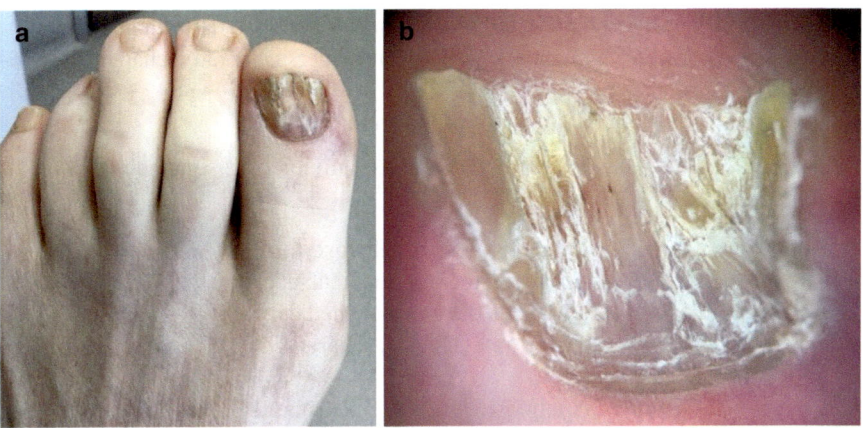

Fig. 41.1 (**a, b**) Sarcoidosis of the left hallux nail demonstrating concavity with longitudinal splitting and erythematous-violaceous discoloration. (Credit: manuscript authors Yim et al.)

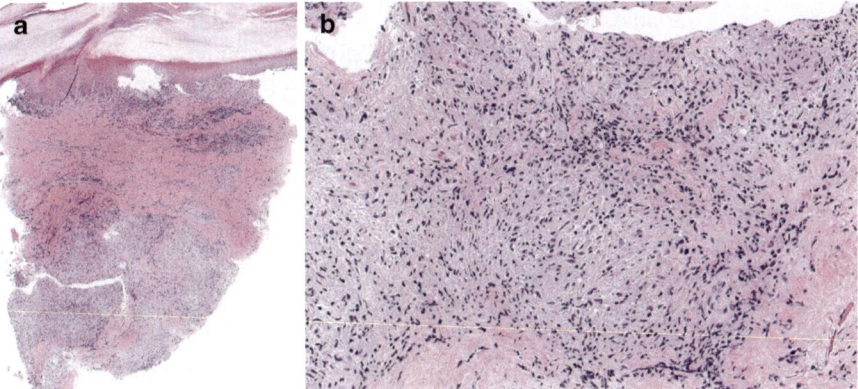

Fig. 41.2 Ill-formed non-necrotizing granulomata with some "naked" granulomas consistent with sarcoidosis shown under punch biopsy of the left hallux nail (hematoxylin and eosin stain); (**a**) magnification ×3, (**b**) magnification ×15. (Credit: manuscript authors Yim et al.)

Based on the Case Description and the Photographs, What Is Your Diagnosis?

Our diagnosis: Sarcoidosis of the nail.
Relevant differential diagnoses: Lichen planus, amyloidosis, squamous cell carcinoma, onychomycosis.

Diagnosis

Correct diagnosis: Sarcoidosis

Discussion

Sarcoidosis is a granulomatous disease often known as the "great imitator" due to its broad and variable clinical presentations of unknown etiology [1–3]. Nail involvement in sarcoidosis is rare and typically presents with nonspecific findings, such as subungual hyperkeratosis, onycholysis, longitudinal ridges, splinter hemorrhages, clubbing, and/or discoloration. [4–7] Nail sarcoidosis has been associated with chronic systemic illness and is often associated with underlying bony involvement, with a previous review of 33 sarcoid nail cases reporting 20 cases that underwent radiographic imaging showed with 17 cases showing the simultaneous presence of nail and underlying osseous sarcoidosis. [4] Physicians should be aware that nail sarcoidosis typically involves osseous abnormalities of associated digit, but lack of abnormalities can occur, as demonstrated in our patient case of longitudinal splitting and erythematous-violaceous discoloration in the left hallux with absent underlying osseous involvement. Since the clinical presentation for nail sarcoidosis varies widely and unfortunately findings are nonspecific, performing nail biopsy is recommended to assist with diagnosis and guide treatment and management. Furthermore, nail involvement in sarcoidosis warrants a thorough evaluation for underlying cutaneous and systemic manifestations.

Key Points

- Nail involvement is a rare presenting sign of chronic systemic illness in sarcoidosis which is usually associated with underlying osseous abnormalities.
- Although nail findings for sarcoidosis can be nonspecific, a nail biopsy can be helpful in diagnosing sarcoidosis and can guide management.

Acknowledgements The patient in this manuscript have given informed consent to publication of their case details.

Funding Sources None.

Conflicts of Interest The authors have no conflict of interest to disclose.

Reprint Requests Elizabeth Yim, MD, MPH.

Statement on Prior Publication The authors state that this manuscript is not under consideration by any other journal and has not been previously published elsewhere.

References

1. Gerke AK. Treatment of sarcoidosis: a multidisciplinary approach. Front Immunol. 2020;11:545413.
2. Santoro F, Sloan SB. Nail dystrophy and bony involvement in chronic sarcoidosis. J Am Acad Dermatol. 2009;60(6):1050–2.
3. Karadağ AS, Parish LC. Sarcoidosis: a great imitator. Clin Dermatol. 2019;37(3):240–54.
4. Momen SE, Al-Niaimi F. Sarcoid and the nail: review of the literature. Clin Exp Dermatol. 2013;38(2):119–24. quiz 125.
5. Noriega L, Criado P, Gabbi T, Avancini J, Di Chiacchio N. Nail sarcoidosis with and without systemic involvement: report of two cases. Skin Appendage Disord. 2015;1(2):87–90.
6. Fernandez-Faith E, McDonnell J. Cutaneous sarcoidosis: differential diagnosis. Clin Dermatol. 2007;25(3):276–87.
7. Lipner SR. Nail disorders: diagnosis and management. Dermatol Clin. 2021;39(2):xi.

Chapter 42
Lightening-Storm Periungual Capillaries in Patient with Complex Regional Pain Syndrome Type 1

Sarah Alenezi and Martin N. Zaiac

Abstract This is a case using dermoscopy and onychoscopy to highlight a pattern of periungual capillaries and facial vessels which we have call "Lightening Storm".

These were noted in a patient with Complex Regional Syndrome. The similarity in the vessels both on the cheeks and the periungual area were noted.

To our knowledge this pattern of vasculature has not been described.

Keywords Lightening storm · Dermoscopy · Onychoscopy · Regional pain syndrome · Periungual

Clinical Case

A 75-year-old male presented to the dermatology clinic. He reported a 10-year history of complex regional pain syndrome (CRPS) that developed after experiencing trauma to the proximal left lateral forearm. He is on analgesics due to constant pain in the forearm and hand, The patient's medical history reveals a prior diagnosis of keratoacanthoma in the proximal segment of the posterior forearm. Moreover, he has a documented history of past drug addiction,

S. Alenezi
Dr. Phillip Frost Department of Dermatology and Cutaneous Surgery, University of Miami Miller School of Medicine, Miami, FL, USA

M. N. Zaiac (✉)
Department of Dermatology, Herbert Wertheim Collage of Medicine, Florida International University, Miami, FL, USA

Greater Miami Skin and Laser Center, Mount Sinai Medical Center, Miami, FL, USA

© The Author(s), under exclusive license to Springer Nature Switzerland AG 2025
A. Tosti et al. (eds.), *Clinical Cases in Nail Disorders*, Clinical Cases in Dermatology, https://doi.org/10.1007/978-3-031-88642-3_42

smoking, and alcohol consumption. He has sought medical attention at the dermatology clinic multiple times due to friction, swelling, and discomfort in the forearm and hand. During this visit, the patient exhibited erythema, stinging and a burning sensation on the face (Fig. 42.1), which exacerbated his preexisting rosacea condition.

During the physical examination of the face, vascular changes were observed in the cheeks (Fig. 42.2), suggesting neurologic rosacea. In the forearm examination, linear skin damage consistent with friction and mechanical trauma was noted in the proximal segment of the lateral left forearm, with no muscle wasting or joint stiffness. The patient denied experiencing any skin bleeding or itching. Additionally, nail examination revealed longitudinal erythronychia and onycholysis, with the proximal and lateral nail folds appearing normal with no atrophy noticed. Using a Fotofinder, photographs were taken to capture detailed images of the nail folds, upon onychoscopy, an irregular pattern of capillary loops was discovered, characterized by oversized and tortuous vessels, forming a striking "lightning-storm" configuration (Figs. 42.3 and 42.4). Furthermore, there was a noticeable deviation from the typical parallel motif. Alongside these observations, pinpoint loops were observed and certain regions of the proximal nail fold. These distinctive features were evident across all finger nail units.

Laboratory testing revealed a complete blood count (CBC) and comprehensive metabolic panel (CMP) within the normal range, plain film radiography, and MRI were unremarkable.

Fig. 42.1 Lateral side of the face with erythematous flushing, visible blood vessels in the cheeks area

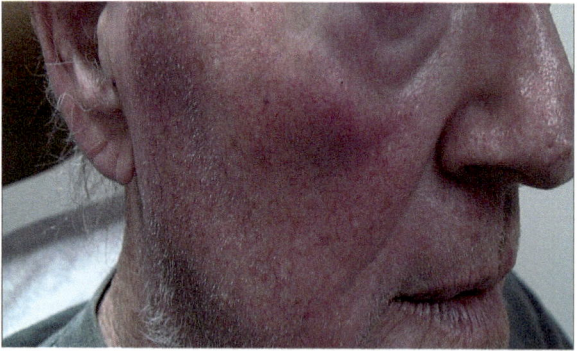

Fig. 42.2 Dermoscopic examination on the lateral side of the face, appearance of a network of tortuous and dilated blood vessels that resemble lightning bolts. a "lightning-storm" appearance

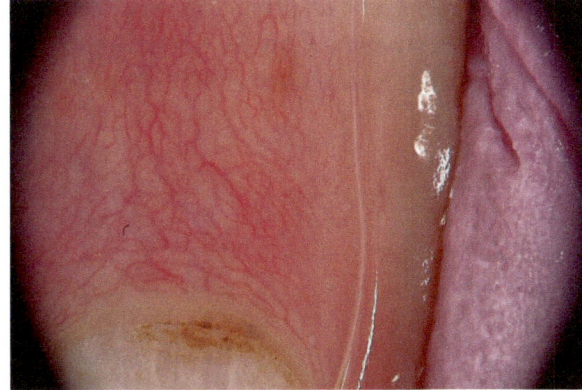

Fig. 42.3 Onychoscopy examination on the nail folds, the presence of tortuous capillaries a "lightning-storm" appearance

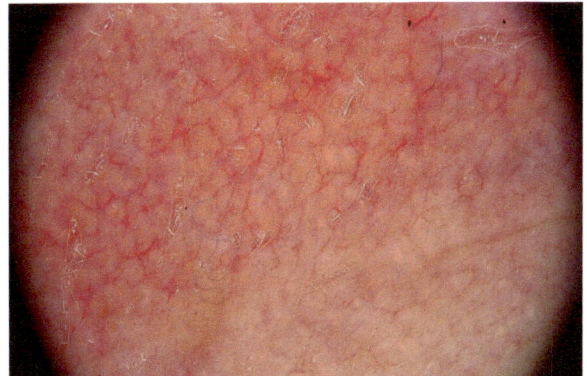

Fig. 42.4 Onychoscopy examination on the nail folds twisted and elongated blood vessels forming "lightning-storm" appearance, pinpoint loops observed

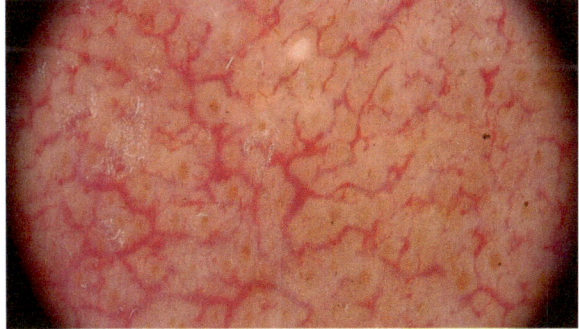

Based on the Case Description and the Photographs, What Is Nail Manifestations Can Be Associated with Complex Regional Pain Syndrome (CRPS)?

A. Onychomycosis
B. Periungual warts
C. Psoriasis of the nail
D. Vascular changes in the nail fold
E. Kolionychia

Answer

D. Vascular change in the nail fold

In this case, the patient presented with onycholysis and longitudinal erythronychia, Additionally, vascular changes forming lightening -storm appearance were observed in the nail fold using onychoscopy, indicating abnormalities in the blood vessels within the nail area. These findings suggest possible underlying vascular and inflammatory conditions that could be contributing to these nail manifestations.

Also in this case patient complain of other dermatologic manifestation: neurologic rosacea affecting the face (flushing, tingling, burning).

Discussion

In 1994, the International Association for the Study of Pain (IASP) introduced the term "Complex Regional Pain Syndrome" (CRPS) in the Classification of Chronic Pain, distinguishing it into two types. CRPS type 1, previously known as reflex sympathetic dystrophy (RSD), occurs without a definite nerve injury, whereas CRPS type 2, formerly known as causalgia, occurs with a documented nerve injury. Both types typically develop after trauma [1]. Pain is the primary concern in complex regional pain syndrome (CRPS), and it often exceeds what would be expected based on the severity of the initial injury. This pain can be persistent and may not respond adequately to traditional pain medications, including narcotics [2], Recognizing complex regional pain syndrome (CRPS) in a dermatologic setting is vital, as skin abnormalities can be the only signs observed during examination. Furthermore, these skin findings may become more prominent as the disease advances to later stages [3]. Neurogenic rosacea refers to the presence of rosacea symptoms in individuals with complex regional pain syndrome (CRPS) [4], nail manifestations in CRPS have been observed and documented include Unilateral leukonychia, Beau's lines, nailfold swelling, and nail clubbing, trachonychia [5], whitlow like presentation [6]. These nail abnormalities can occur as a result of the condition, indicating possible underlying vascular and inflammatory changes associated with (CRPS) [6], in this case when performing onychoscopy on the nail folds, a "lightning-storm" appearance may be observed. This term describes the visual appearance of a network of tortuous and dilated blood vessels that resemble lightning bolts. This finding suggests significant vascular abnormalities within the nail fold, vascular changes in complex regional pain syndrome (CRPS) have been investigated using different methods and have shown varied results [7]. Early studies indicated increased blood flow in affected extremities, suggesting enhanced perfusion. However, capillaroscopy studies found lower capillary blood cell velocity (CBV) and laser Doppler flux (LDF) values in the nail fold skin of CRPS patients compared to controls, despite similar skin temperatures [8]. These discrepancies may be attributed to the disease stage and the specific layers of skin being measured for blood flow. In a study by Kurvers et al., they investigated the stages of reflex sympathetic dystrophy (RSD) and their impact on skin blood flow [9]. CRPS was divided into three stages, characterized by different sensations: chronic warmth (stage I), intermittent warmth and cold (stage II), and chronic cold (stage III) [9].

The study revealed that total skin blood flow was increased in stage I but decreased in stages II and III compared to controls. Nutritive skin blood flow was also lower in stages II and III. Interestingly, capillary diameter and density in the nail fold did not differ between controls and patients, and they did not change with the duration of the syndrome. However, capillary diameter was larger in stage III compared to stage II and possibly stage I [9].

These findings differ from Tosti et al.'s study, where they observed a vascular nodule with proliferating capillary vessels and inflammation in the proximal nail fold, suggesting that vasoproliferation contributes to the increased blood flow seen in the early inflammatory stage of CRPS-I [6], Recognizing and diagnosing complex regional pain syndrome (CRPS) can be challenging due to a wide range of reported clinical characteristics and a nonspecific clinical presentation. However, nail fold capillaroscopy holds potential as a useful and accessible tool for evaluating patients with CRPS,

In summary, the patient presents with several dermatologic manifestations, including longitudinal erythronychia and vascular changes in the nail fold observed through onychoscopy with unique lightning-storm" appearance. Along with these findings, the patient also complains of neurologic rosacea, it's important to identify the dermatologic manifestations as they can serve as important diagnostic indicators and aid in monitoring the progress of CRPS-I, even when other physical examination findings are minimal or absent.

Key Points

- "Lightning-storm" pattern, observed in individuals with complex regional pain syndrome (CRPS) provide important diagnostic clues and insights into the impact of CRPS on nail health.
- lightning-storm" pattern refers to the presence of striking vascular abnormalities characterized by a network of tortuous and dilated blood vessels resembling lightning bolts. This finding can be indicative of the vascular dysfunction associated with CRPS and can aid in the diagnosis and assessment of the condition.
- Nail fold capillaroscopy has shown potential as a valuable and easily accessible tool for evaluating patients with complex regional pain syndrome (CRPS). This diagnostic technique allows for the examination of the capillaries in the nail fold, providing information about microvascular abnormalities and potential changes associated with CRPS
- In some cases of complex regional pain syndrome type 1 (CRPS-I), dermatologic changes may be the only physical examination findings.

References

1. Misidou C, Papagoras C. Complex regional pain syndrome: an update. Mediterr J Rheumatol. 2019;30(1):16–25.
2. Field J. Complex regional pain syndrome: a review. J Hand Surg Eur Vol. 2013;38(6):616–26.
3. Kabani R, Brassard A. Dermatological findings in early detection of complex regional pain syndrome. JAMA Dermatol. 2014;150(6):640–2.
4. Schram AM, James WD. Neurogenic rosacea treated with endoscopic thoracic sympathectomy. Arch Dermatol. 2012;148(2):270–1.
5. Pucevich B, Spencer L, English JC III. Unilateral trachyonychia in a patient with reflex sympathetic dystrophy. J Am Acad Dermatol. 2008;58(2):320–2.
6. Tosti A, et al. Reflex sympathetic dystrophy with prominent involvement of the nail apparatus. J Am Acad Dermatol. 1993;29(5):865–8.
7. Kozin F, et al. The reflex sympathetic dystrophy syndrome (RSDS): III. Scintigraphic studies, further evidence for the therapeutic efficacy of systemic corticosteroids, and proposed diagnostic criteria. Am J Med. 1981;70(1):23–30.
8. Rosen L, et al. Skin microvascular circulation in the sympathetic dystrophies evaluated by videophotometric capillaroscopy and laser Doppler fluxmetry. Eur J Clin Investig. 1988;18(3):305–8.
9. Kurvers H, et al. Reflex sympathetic dystrophy: evolution of microcirculatory disturbances in time. Pain. 1995;60(3):333–40.